HAIR TODAY, MORE TOMORROW

How to Keep your Hair On...
the ULTIMATE Guide for Women.

Sara G Allison
RGN MIT WTS EHRS

World leading Harley
Street Trichologist

Orders: Please contact +44 20 7299 0383

You can also order via the e mail address
mail@hairlossconsultant.co.uk

ISBN: 978-0-9935540-0-1

First published 2016 by Hair Today More Tomorrow Limited.

Printed in Great Britain for Hair Today More Tomorrow Ltd by Bell & Bain Ltd, 303 Burnfield Road, Thornliebank, Glasgow G46 7UQ

CONTENTS

SARA G. ALLISON

Sara G. Allison is not only a world-leading Harley Street trichologist, but she is also a registered nurse with extensive senior experience at prestigious London hospitals and university practices, giving her a unique perspective and experience in woman's health.

As the founder of Hair Today More Tomorrow, she has created a range of products and services which have been praised by celebrities, Marie Claire, Prima, The Telegraph, The Times and more.

Sara began her career specialising in women's health at Queen Charlotte's and Chelsea Hospital. She later went on to work as a senior nurse at the world renowned Elizabeth Garret Anderson hospital for women.

Here she obtained further qualifications in reproductive and sexual health, which lead her to develop an expertise in the complex issues involving female hair loss.

As a qualified trichologist, Sara decided to expand her medical knowledge, and became a senior nurse advisor for the NHS Direct, then a nurse practitioner in general practice, linked to University College London.

In 1999 she decided to start her own practice and focus solely on trichology at Harley Street where she discovered a strong link between nutrition, hair, and skin.

In fact, she found herself recommending lots of different products to treat hair loss, but she wasn't completely happy with the results. So she decided to work with a team of scientists to produce a range of high quality hair and anti-ageing products that; boost regular hair growth and shine; produce radiant and refined skin; and develop strong, shiny nails.

Sara is adamant about keeping up to date with the latest advances in research. She incorporates this knowledge into the advice she gives her clients and the media. Sara is regularly featured in the UK media as an expert trichologist.

To book an appointment with Sara, please visit hairlossconsultant.co.uk

PREFACE

As the gynaecology ward sister, it was my role to partake in the doctor's rounds, where the patients were nodding politely while the consultants were telling them in length all about their conditions. The doctors left the ward feeling confident that they'd done their job, but I would turn and see the perplexed looks on the faces of their patients, and I just knew they actually didn't understand a word of it! So I would return to their bedsides and interpret doctor's terminology for them into simple English; it was a common scenario in those days, but I had a knack for converting complex subjects. Move forward in time to now and I'm a trichologist with the very niche speciality of hair loss in women! Therefore, I hope you appreciate the way I've written this book with appropriate bullet points aimed at answering your questions, in as clear a way as possible for you.

WHO THIS BOOK IS FOR...

Your hair is really the only thing you can change about your physical appearance, it's a form of expression of your identity and if you lose a sense of control over it; then it's not surprising that it has the potential to affect your mood and self-esteem.

You may feel terribly self-conscious, ashamed and think everyone is noticing your thinning hair; this gives you low self-esteem, and confidence levels. Some women have complained how they feel they've been turned down for jobs due to their hair and that they have lack of confidence in themselves so their work suffers. Relationships can also break down due to your anxiety and you may be withdrawing from physical intimacy and avoiding social contact too. The whole issue could therefore be causing you complete isolation and depression.

With this isolation you have created, you probably rarely discuss your hair loss with anyone and female hair loss has not been widely accepted by society; so when women initially see me they are so distressed at the release of their tension, that they often breakdown in tears. Hair loss in women is so stressful that I've frequently had clients that say it's THE most stressful thing that's happened to them, they've felt even worse about their hair than when they had been diagnosed with life threatening illnesses.

Hopefully, you're reading this early on, before you've reached these stages of despair and just want to know what you can do to improve your hair.

I should therefore start, by explaining for my international readers the phrase "Keep your hair on!" is actually a common English idiom used to encourage someone that is getting very stressed and upset about something to take stock of the situation and calm down!

I totally understand this is how you'll be feeling, so please read this guide carefully and you will find my reassuring revelations, that you have never known before and will indeed help you well on the way to keeping your hair on…

HAIR A REFLECTION OF FERTILITY

We have evolved with the concept that women with glossy, lustrous, long hair are the most attractive. Subconsciously this is due to hair being a reflection of fertility and it has been shown that men's top attribute of physical attractiveness when looking for a partner is 'shiny, full hair'; hence hair projects youth, health, femininity and sexual desire. It is no wonder then, that the experience of thinning hair at any age is bound to be anxiety provoking for you.

Whilst society fully accepts that men suffer from hair loss, as a woman you are likely to be embarrassed to admit to hair loss as you may consider it socially unacceptable. Likewise, as a trichologist people automatically assume my clients are predominately middle aged, bald men. However, the majority of my clients are actually women. There is no upper limit to age when it comes to being a woman and worrying about your hair and I even have clients in their nineties; if you are a woman that cares about good grooming this doesn't change as you age and you will continue to care about your appearance. Of course we are living longer and are being more image conscious than before, therefore your hair at any age is of paramount importance even well past your fertile years.

It was found that over half of women with hair loss find themselves making excuses not to be sexual with their partners as a result of feeling less attractive. Therefore their partners often consequently suffer physically and emotionally from their hair loss. Of those without a partner 96% said having hair loss impacted them meeting someone new.

As a Trichologist my speciality within the field is hair loss in women, and in gynaecology it was fertility; it is my opinion that, whatever is good for your hair is also good for your fertility and interesting, just as hair loss is increasing so are infertility rates!

A GROWING PROBLEM

People still don't really appreciate how common it really is and you may think you're the only one suffering, especially as you wouldn't necessarily notice just by looking around; because for a woman it's quite easy to change your hair style to disguise any areas of thinning. Unfortunately, though female hair loss is incredibly common and one in three women over twenty five years old suffer from hair loss; and this seems to be continually increasing, with a doctors survey saying they that they had noticed a 64% increase in their patients over the last five years. I feel this is just the tip of the iceberg though as it's such a taboo subject and women are suffering in silence; I compare talking about hair loss for a woman, to a man talking about his impotency! When it's happening to you, it's one of those rare subjects that you just don't mention, however I strongly hope that will change and that women become more open about it, as then you and others will find the necessary support!

So with that in mind I hope you find the rest of this guide very enlightening to know you're far from alone…

WHY AM I LOSING MY HAIR?

I usually find that there are a combination of reasons! Just one of these by itself, may or may not make much noticeable difference, but when you have two or more potential causes together then the effects are really magnified. I have listed the most common ones that I come across in my practice...

Stress

Stress is the word that many people use when they are describing how the demands of their life seems to be becoming too great for them to cope with, and many of us would like to find ways to gain some control over it. Emotional stress can result from any significant life changes and crises. Injury, surgery and illness can cause physical stress. Unfortunately most of us are leading more emotionally stressful lives and this stress can either be responsible for many of the hair loss conditions or at least exacerbate them.

The ability to cope with stress varies from person to person and what one person finds stressful may not be a problem for another. Whilst many of us suffer with stress at times in our day to day lives, long term stress is known to be bad for our health and can trigger hair loss too.

How does stress cause hair loss?

Stress has major physiologic impacts on our body, it causes inflammation in the body and this is one of the major factors of hair loss. When our body is stressed (also known as the stress response) it produces and releases toxins that are dangerous in excess. When one imbalance occurs in the body, there is a knock on effect elsewhere. Adrenals produce the stress hormone cortisol and when you produce more of this, it will lower the female hormone progesterone; which can have implications on female pattern hair loss. Sometimes, blood supply to hair follicles is compromised, which results in hair falling out because growth cannot be sustained. Sometimes you will notice the effects of excessive shedding immediately or just thinning about three to four months after a stressful episode.

I'm not sure if I'm stressed, how can I tell?

The signs of stress vary from person to person but here are some of the most common ones, you may only have a couple of them.

Physical signs:

Hair loss, headaches, muscle tension or pain, digestive problems like IBS or acid reflux or ulcers, bladder problems, fatigue, sleep problems, excessive sweating, dizziness, breathlessness or palpitations dry mouth, tingling in body, sexual problems

Emotional symptoms;

Irritability, feeling anxious or tense, low mood, apathy, low self- esteem.

Reactions;

Temper outbursts, excessive drinking or smoking, changes in eating habits, withdrawing from usual activities, becoming unreasonable, forgetfulness or clumsiness, rushing around.

What may have caused the stress in the first place?

Some things that happen in your life can be stressful particularly life changes. If you have had one or more of the following life events occurring over the last year your hair loss may be a result of stress;

divorce or relationship breakdown, legal issues, getting married, pregnancy, health problems, difficulty conceiving, financial problems, change in living conditions, building renovations, disagreements with friends or family, problems at work, e.g, loss of employment, lack of job security, several jobs, no satisfaction at work, unemployment, new job, major changes at work, partner stops or begins work, problems with neighbours/noise, family gatherings for holidays/Christmas and lastly bereavement for family or friends. And don't underestimate the emotional effects of grieving for a beloved pets too. I have several clients that have suffered hair loss from the distress of losing a pet. I have even experienced this myself. One lady had lost her two elderly parents and her aunt in the space of few months, but she also lost her cat at the same time and she was reluctant to admit for fear of being judged that losing her cat was the one she really couldn't cope with and no doubt was the one that caused her hair loss.

Of course having hair loss in itself is a major stress! And the thing that started the stress in the first instance may well have been resolved and now you're simply stressed about your hair!

So how can stress be relieved?

As part of my consultation I frequently do a little counselling too and then together discuss ways that an individual may be able to alleviate their stress. This really is so important and a huge part of hair loss cure, as if the stress remains present then recovery is very difficult.

Fortunately, there are many things you can do to relieve the damaging excess of the stress hormone cortisol and simultaneously improve your overall health. Studies show that the first step in tackling stress is to become aware that it is a problem for you- half the battle is admitting it!

- Identify the stress and then take control of any of your areas in your life that are causing stress.

- Focus on the present, depression occurs from dwelling on the past and anxiety from worrying about the future, but if you stay present in the moment this really helps.

- Take time off for a holiday.

- Communication is very important if stress if related to relationships with others or just to get support from your family or friends.

- If work is the problem, identify what needs addressing and weigh up your options, and what can you do to change the situation, could you retrain or work in a different area or change companies, or could you get more support from your manager or delegate to others?

- Keep a sensible work life balance, i.e. don't over work yourself and take time for relaxation and to enjoy yourself.

- Seek professional help, if you have tried these things and still your stress is a problem.

Proven ways promoting feel good endorphins and counterbalance/relieve stress are:

- Exercise three to five times a week, i.e. at least thirty minutes and keep to it in moderation only.
- Meditation. Frequent mediation will lead to an emotional, physical and psychological balance. It's easy to do in any quiet spot and you don't need any equipment.
- Balanced nutrition is another key to reducing stress levels. If your diet is rich in nutrients and vitamins, you will be less tired, more focused, and thus more capable of coping with stress.
- Regular massages
- Stroking pets.
- Practising mindfulness.
- Physical intimacy
- Spending time with 'quality' friends.
- Spend time in nature wherever possible.
- Relaxation techniques, such as deep breathing and/or muscular tensing and stretching.

Medications

These often have numerous side effects and so much of the population are taking prescribed medication nowadays, plus the older you are the more likely this is the case. There is a statistic that more than 90% of conventional drugs only work in 30-50% of people, as individuals all react differently to different stimuli, therefore there is no hard and fast rule, just discuss your medication with your prescribing doctor.

Side effects of medications can cause alopecia or excessive hair loss and particular common culprits are;

- Statins which are used to lower cholesterol
- Cox inhibitors which are NSAIDs (non steroidal anti-inflammatories) painkillers such Aspirin, Ibuprofen/Advil and Naproxen.

- Anti-depressants.

- Nicotine replacement therapy.

- Beta blockers for high blood pressure.

- Warfarin for thinning the blood.

- Protein pump inhibitors (PPIs) and antacids e.g. Lansporazole, Omeprazole, Ranitidine, Gaviscon, as they can affect the intrinsic factor in your stomach, so you could get low vitamin B12, which is one of the key vitamins for hair. They also lower the stomach acid, which will impair the absorption of nutrients. Mastic gum, slippery elm and glutamine are good natural alternatives for gastric symptoms.

Vitamin D Deficiency

There is a worldwide epidemic of vitamin D deficiency due to modern lifestyles which mean we spend more time indoors or using transportation rather than outdoors being exposed to unhindered UVB sun rays. Those that are lucky enough to get some sun exposure, then actually block these necessary UVB rays by using sun screen!

Vitamin D is vital not only for your hair and skin, but for your whole body therefore I urge those of you living in European and North American latitudes to increase vital vitamin D absorption with optimal sun exposure. We need the UVB rays to be at the right level and this is achieved between the months of April to October. If you live in the southern hemisphere then it will be the opposite months of October though to April. Nearer the equator (where we all originally evolved from) we can obtain vitamin D from the sun all year round.

Research on vitamin D shows that it preserves and protects DNA changes, thereby helping cell growth and anti-ageing. Hair follicles do have vitamin D receptor sites and in my experience there is a correlation with hair growth/ loss and therefore, I like to monitor all my clients blood results and 'prescribe' an individual dosage of supplements as necessary.

Windows and sun screen block the UVB rays necessary for vitamin D production, therefore, whenever possible, ensure 20 minutes of sun on bare skin between hours of 10am and 3pm. You may wish to put sun screen on your face though, just to help maintain your complexion.

If you are fortunate enough to have the time and money then winter holidays to escape to the sun nearer the equator or on your opposite hemisphere will be well worth it for your mind, body and hair!

In addition to getting the 'safe' amounts of sun whenever possible, I also highly recommend taking Hair Today More Tomorrow Multi & Omegas, which as well as many other nutrients contains 2,000 i.u of vitamin D. This formulation includes essential fatty acids (Omegas 3,6 & 9) and vitamin K2 and it's important to take all of these together for best absorption.

Dieting

Isn't it good to be slim?

Society's obsession with being thin leads women to eat less as they try to imitate the skinny frames of celebrities. It is good to be the correct weight for your height, but dieting, especially extreme dieting that deprives the body of vital nutrients and vitamins is a known and proven cause of hair loss. In fact, extreme dieting sometimes referred to as "fads" is the leading cause of hair loss and it's very common for me to see women that have been on diets. So whilst it's commendable to quickly shedding some pounds, you are likely shedding your hair as well.

In today's society, it is so much more difficult to get the right nutrients in our diet, plus the media pressure on women to stay thin, often means that you are;

- Regularly on diets.
- Simply don't eat enough to get all the nutrients.
- Not eating the right foods
- Skip meals, either because they're too busy or think it helps to reduce calories.

Why is dieting bad for my hair?

Extreme diets often focus on reducing the amount of calories and fat you consume, but don't always take into account the importance of a nutrient-rich diet. When the body is deprived of important nutrients, hair shafts are weakened, which causes hair breakage and slows down the rate of hair re-growth. The natural hair growth cycle is disrupted so that hair follicles that were growing are converted prematurely to the cycle's shedding and resting stages.

Some experts are sceptical that there is a connection between hair loss and poor diet. What convinces you that there is one?

There is a wealth of research evidence linking nutrition to hair loss. Plus I commonly see ladies in my practice that are suffering hair loss as a result of dieting and weight loss.

What are your top 'dieting' tips for hair?

- DO NOT 'DIET'!

- Eating IS good for you and your hair, of course just ensure you eat the correct foods and a nutrient rich diet; follow my nutrition advice chapter.

- Take Hair Today More Tomorrow Multi & Omegas as a complement, not as a replacement, to your balanced, nutrient-rich diet.

- Lose weight slowly and no more than one to two pounds a week, as toxins are stored in fat cells so when overweight people go on a detox or lose weight, they feel terrible due to all the toxins being released and hair loss can occur as a result of the release of these toxins too.

- Detox before trying to lose weight; as toxins that are held in your fat cells will be released into your blood stream during weight loss which can have side effects of hair loss and lethargy. You need to consume essential fats to detox.

- Don't skip meals.

- Avoid a low fat diet. Sugar NOT fat is what makes people fat and if you have a low fat diet it's impossible to lose weight.

- You need eat at least three small protein meals per day

- If you are having difficulty putting an end to extreme dieting, you may be suffering from an eating disorder. Contact a health professional immediately. There are many treatment options and support groups available to help you.

- Just as I encourage you not to focus on your hair! Please do not focus on your weight either! Just look after yourself and simply follow my guide and your natural weight will happen without you realising it, just as you and your hair will start noticing the benefits too.

- De-Stress as much as possible! Studies have shown the levels of the stress hormone cortisol go up when dieting, so this backs up the fact that dieting is stressful! Not only that but cortisol predisposes to fat deposits around the middle. Stress can impair absorption of nutrients and increase your body's demand for more nutrient dense foods. All things in moderation as long as you're good 80% of the time. The most important thing is to de-stress! Enjoy life and good food, nutritious food is actually really delicious!

- If you really feel that you are unable to lose weight despite following my nutrition advice and exercising then please see your doctor for blood tests to check you don't have any underlying medical conditions causing weight problems.

- Dieting causes nutrition depletion. Studies show that those taking supplements whilst dieting had better weight loss and were more likely to be able to maintain better hair health. Therefore, I would advise you take Hair Today More Tomorrow Multi & Omegas which also contain the necessary essential fats.

Smoking

Is there evidence that smoking can speed up the process of losing hair quicker as we age?

Yes there are studies that indicate smoking can take its toll on your hair with generalised hair thinning, but it can also accelerate hair loss in weaker areas like the front and top or result in a receding hair line or a wider parting.

How can smoking increase ageing in hair?

Smoking has inflammatory and oxidative effects and can deplete the body of essential nutrients, such as zinc, B vitamins, carotene, magnesium, calcium and vitamin C. These factors all contribute to DNA damage at the hair follicles which accelerates the ageing process.

Are there any other points that need to be flagged up as regards smoking and our hair?

The negative effects of smoking on your hair are not limited just to increased hair thinning, but also loss of lustre, lifelessness and accelerated greying hair.

Does smoking also have an impact on the hair of a younger smoker if so why?

Yes these effects can be noticed at any age. This is because depletion of essential nutrients and oxidative stress can affect you regardless of age.

If someone stops smoking is the damage done, or can the negative impact be reversed?

It's definitely worth stopping smoking to see the negative impacts halted and sometimes even reversed, but to maximise the chance of this happening I would advise taking a good quality multi vitamin and mineral, such as Hair Today More Tomorrow Multi & Omegas as this contains all the anti-oxidants and other essentials that would have been depleted. www.hairtodaymoretomorrow.co.uk

Main Gynaecological Causes Of Hair Loss

Infertility

With my background as a senior gynaecology nurse specialist and then becoming a trichologist people often are surprised at the 'jump' as they perceive hair and gynaecology to be such different disciplines, however because of my unique interest in the two fields, I have actually found my own strong correlation with all manner of gynaecological disorders and hair loss. In fact as a Trichologist my speciality within the field is hair loss in women, and in gynaecology it was fertility; it is my opinion that, whatever is good for your hair is also good for your fertility and interesting, just as hair loss is increasing so are infertility rates! Therefore infertility is not so much a cause but it definitely goes hand in hand with hair loss. It is encouraging, that many of my clients become pregnant whilst following their bespoke treatment plans that I provide for them

Hormonal contraceptives

Hormonal contraceptives contain oestrogen and progesterone and there are many different brands. The component that changes the most in each brand is the type of progesterone. Some are much more 'hair friendly' than others and as everyone is an individual, what may affect one woman in one way will effect another in a different way. However there are some that are more likely to cause hair loss than others and some will actually be beneficial for your hair. If you notice hair loss when you stop taking a hormonal contraceptive this shedding usually should settle after 4 months. Contraceptive injections only contain progesterone and these types are more likely to cause hair loss, however an unwanted pregnancy can have profound effects therefore if you are thinking of stopping you must discuss this with your doctor.

Pregnancy

Due to the increased levels of progesterone and oestrogen during pregnancy, women often have thicker, more luxurious hair and never looked healthier. Unfortunately though, hair begins to fall out about three to four months either after childbirth or the cessation of breast feeding. Not to worry, though as this is only temporary shedding, but if your hair does not return to its original condition after a few more months then see a doctor for some blood tests.

Polycystic ovaries

This is a hormonal condition that women can have, from their late teens to their early forties. This can cause hirsutism which is excessive body hair and hair loss in female pattern i.e. thinning on the top and front. Other symptoms could also be greasy hair & skin, with acne and difficulty losing weight. Polycystic ovaries causes women to produce greater amounts of testosterone therefore this can appear like the typical 'menopausal type' female pattern hair loss but in younger women. This should be diagnosed initially with blood tests then pelvic scans to look for cysts on your ovaries and if they find multiple small cysts then PCOS would be diagnosed and doctors would usually prescribe a particular anti-androgenic contraceptive pill and often other prescribed medications too.

Menopause

Menopause is a time in a women's life when her menstrual cycle ends and the sex hormone levels start to fall. However, for approximately five years before the menopause occurs there is a period of time called the peri-menopause, where hormone levels are beginning to change and women can often blame their hair loss on this. Menopause has commonly been described as an oestrogen deficiency disease which has led to the widespread promotion of HRT drugs. However, contrary to popular belief promoted by pharmaceutical advertising, oestrogen levels do not slump at menopause but merely drop about three per cent a year over the average five year menopausal period. Symptoms at this time are often due to relatively low levels of the other female sex hormone progesterone and there does appear to be some relation of hair thinning to lowering testosterone levels too! Many of my clients are in the menopause age range!

Some women who take HRT, find their hair density improves. However, I have certainly seen many ladies experiencing hair loss after starting HRT. With this in mind I do not advise taking HRT just to thicken your hair, unless you also have other menopausal symptoms that need treating. If you do wish to start HRT, ask to be prescribed one that has more positive reports for hair.

However in most instances menopausal symptoms can be helped by regulating hormones naturally by:

- Following my nutrition recommendations. (see separate chapter)
- Quit refined sugar in all its forms.
- Reduce alcohol to a minimum.
- De-stress as much as possible.
- Ensure healthy gut flora by taking a probiotic.
- Balance essential fatty acids.
- Take Hair Today More Tomorrow Multi & Omegas a premier quality multi containing essential fatty acids and probiotics to aid gut health.
- If symptoms don't improve, then seeing a medical herbalist may be beneficial, as they may 'prescribe' a herbal supplement. *50% of women relieve menopause symptoms from correct nutrition, supplementation and detoxing, the remainder from seeing a herbalist.*

Heavy or prolonged menstruation.

This can sometimes be as a result from fibroids in your uterus, these are benign growths that, if left untreated and with the subsequent excessive blood loss, you can easily become low in ferritin; which is a protein that stores iron. A deficiency of this is a common cause of hair loss. Iron deficiency can also affect thyroid metabolism, which is yet another cause of hair thinning.

Health Disorders

Although hair thinning may not be thought of as a medical condition, it is actually a fantastic marker of health and the often the very first signs of a dysfunction somewhere else in your body. Therefore blood tests and detailed history taking are very important to identify any underlying problem. Two of the most common problems are thyroid imbalance and irritable bowel syndrome.

Thyroid Imbalance

The thyroid gland produces hormones that control your metabolic rate, which affects every cell in your body. A thyroid disorder is when you produce too much or too little of these hormones and this is called hyperthyroidism or hypothyroidism, depending on if you're producing too much or too little.

Hair loss can be the first sign of a thyroid imbalance, and is the single most established cause in the medical profession. This can be relatively common in women of all ages presenting with hair problems, but more so over the age of fifty. TSH, T4 & T3 are blood tests which play an important role in diagnosing and managing hyper/hypothyroidism. They help your doctor determine the right dosage of medication, both initially and over time. However my professional experience has led me to establish necessary thyroid hormone blood levels for your hair that are very different from the conventional levels for treatment!

Hypothyroidism is more prevalent than hyperthyroidism and occurs six times more frequently in women than in men. Other symptoms of this apart from hair loss can include; anxiety, depression, dry skin, fatigue, intolerance of cold temperatures, weight gain or struggles to lose it, poor memory, muscle stiffness and infertility.

What are the triggers for thyroid imbalance?

- Stress (due to raised cortisol levels)
- Illness
- Weight loss
- Poor nutrition
- Certain medication

Or often triggered at times of hormonal imbalance such as:

- Menopause.
- Pregnancy.
- Excess oestrogen e.g. oral contraceptives.

If you have a thyroid imbalance you are likely to need prescribed medication, therefore please see your doctor. If they say you don't need medication and you are only a little out of balance then there are there natural ways to help restore the balance:

- Follow my nutrition guidance.
- Take Hair Today More Tomorrow Multi & Omegas which contains many of the nutrients including iodine important for regulating your thyroid.
- Deal with stress.
- Deal with any illnesses, especially digestive problems.
- Avoid fluoride and chlorine which block iodine receptors.
- Get adequate sleep and rest.
- Regular and gentle exercise.

Irritable Bowel Syndrome

What is irritable bowel syndrome and who gets it?

Irritable bowel syndrome (IBS) is a common gut disorder. The cause is not completely established, although stress is definitely related and there is a proven link between the gut and the brain. Intolerance to certain foods may play a part in many cases and, it can also occur following gastroenteritis or the use of antibiotics. Symptoms can be quite variable and include abdominal pain, bloating, and sometimes bouts of diarrhoea and/or constipation. Symptoms tend to 'come and go'. There is no 'cure' for IBS, but symptoms can often be eased with treatment. IBS can affect anyone at any age, but it commonly first develops in young adults and teenagers and women are affected more often than men.

How can IBS affect hair health?

You are probably surprised to see a mention of IBS in a book about hair and wonder why I've included it, but this is actually quite a common syndrome and approximately 20% of my clients suffer from IBS symptoms at some stage in their life. Due to this dysfunction of your gut, it makes it more difficult to absorb all the nutrients from your diet, and in particular, zinc, iron and proteins. All of which are important in hair health, therefore deficiencies and associated hair loss can result. Hence it is important to treat any IBS and your nutrient intake and hair should subsequently improve.

What are the treatments for irritable bowel syndrome?

A healthy diet is important for all of us. However, some people with IBS find certain foods in a normal healthy diet can trigger symptoms or make symptoms worse. Therefore it may help to keep a food and lifestyle diary for two to four weeks to monitor symptoms and activities. Note everything that you eat and drink, times that you were stressed, and when you took any formal exercise (regular exercise may also help to ease symptoms). This may identify triggers, such as a food, alcohol, or emotional stresses, and may show if exercise helps to ease or to prevent symptoms. The foods that are most commonly reported to cause IBS symptoms are: wheat, dairy products, rye, barley, caffeine in coffee, tea and cola and onions.

Stress and other emotional factors may trigger symptoms in some people. So, anything that can reduce your level of stress or emotional upset may help. The relationship between the mind, brain, nervous impulses and over-activity of internal organs such as the gut is complex. Some people have found such things as relaxation techniques, stress counselling, cognitive behaviour therapy, psychotherapy, hypnotherapy, and similar therapies useful in controlling symptoms of IBS.

With IBS and hair loss and your poor gut absorption you especially need to optimise the amount of nutrients you are consuming, I would therefore recommend taking Hair Today More Tomorrow Multi & Omegas, which contains a comprehensive range including the most important for gut function, such as zinc, vitamin D, omega 3 and probiotics.

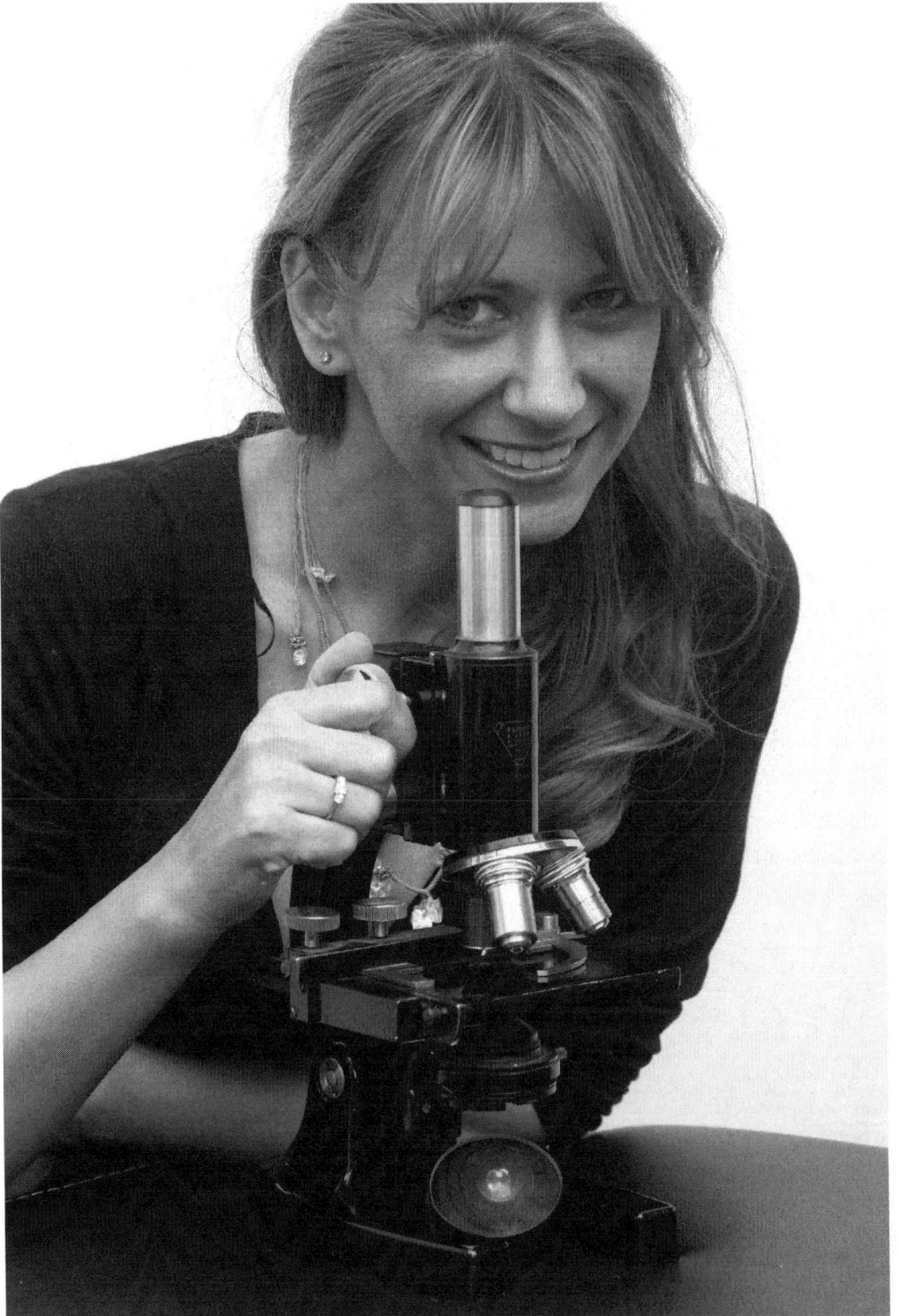

TO UNDERSTAND THE FOLLOWING HAIR & SCALP CONDITIONS YOU SHOULD FIRST KNOW A FEW HAIR BIOLOGY FACTS

Hair loss affects women just as much as men!

Hair is made in tiny pouches in the skin called hair follicles.

Hair grows about 1cm growth per month.

Each scalp hair has a normal 'life cycle'

Hair will grow in the anagen phase for about two to six years, but usually its three to four years.

Each hair will then come to the end of its life and falls out in the telogen shedding phase which lasts about three to four months.

Kenogen is the resting phase after hairs have been released from an empty follicle and this phase comes before the new anagen hair starts to develop. The length of time for this changes and this is the phase where a lot of hair research is ongoing. It is observed more in frequency and duration in both males and females with androgenic alopecia.

The cycle should start again to make a new hair.

Hair follicles should usually be at varying stages of their cycle.

When this balance is disturbed and more hairs are shed than are regrown, alopecia or hair loss results.

At any one time about one in a hundred scalp hairs are at the end of their life ready to fall out, therefore each person sheds hair and regrows hair every day approximately; one hundred hairs if you have a full head of hair. This is why you will commonly find a few hairs on your shoulders, and some hairs fall out each time you wash your hair.

When this balance is disturbed and more hairs are shed than are regrown, hair thinning results.

Both men and women tend to lose both their hair thickness and volume as they age. About one-half of men begin to bald by the time they are 30 years old, and most are either bald or have a balding pattern by age 60.

White 'grey' hairs on older people appear to grow faster than pigmented hair of the younger.

Therefore, it appears the effect of producing pigment prohibits growth.

White hairs can be made to produce pigment again with the right stimulation!

Follicles change shape dramatically with age, they are smooth in a child resulting in straighter hair. They are a variety of shapes in the young adult. At middle age the follicles start stabilising and in old age they go back to smooth again, but then they will be grey instead of pigmented.

Hair loss can become a cosmetic problem when it occurs in the wrong place at the wrong time. True hair loss should be distinguished from damage to the hair shaft, which may cause breakage close to the scalp. This type of damage is most often caused by chemicals like misuse of hair dye.

COMMON HAIR & SCALP CONDITIONS

People are often surprised to hear that there are many different types of hair loss conditions. I have included only the most common conditions here. However, diagnosis can often be difficult and I frequently find that my clients have a couple of conditions together, therefore, the next chapter is only for you to understand what may or may not be happening to you and I urge you not to self-diagnose. I have included a couple of scalp conditions because they are often a precursor to hair loss therefore they need early management. For instance I often see clients that have tolerated scalp psoriasis for around 20 years, but then when they notice they are getting hair loss, suddenly it is an urgent issue for them.

Telogen Effluvium

This condition is by far the most common and often plays a hand in other conditions too, by exacerbating them! In particular this often occurs together with female pattern hair loss. Telogen effluvium is a condition where more than normal amounts of hair fall out. There is a general 'thinning' of the hair. Unlike some other hair and scalp conditions, this one is temporary and completely reversible if you eliminate the cause. However, I have seen clients who have had this condition for over thirty years before seeing me and that's because the cause had previously never been correctly identified and eliminated.

What are the symptoms of telogen effluvium?

An increase in the amount of hair shedding. This is more than normal and most noticeable when you wash your hair. However, your scalp and the remaining hair look healthy. You will not have patches of hair loss (bald patches), but rather a generalised thinning. You can have a more chronic form of telogen effluvium where you don't see the shedding, but the hair gradually gets a diffuse thinning over many years.

Why does telogen effluvium occur?

Changes to the body cause the older hairs to be brought to an end of their life cycle earlier than the usual three to four years, by entering the telogen phase prematurely. Many more hairs than usual are then ready to fall out. It takes three to four months for the affected hairs to fall out after their growth has stopped. After a resting period, new hairs then grow from the hair follicles as usual. A normal pattern and thickness of hair returns within a few months once these new hairs are established and if the cause has been addressed.

Common causes could be;

Stress, sub optimal nutrition, having a baby, stopping breast feeding, major surgery, stopping or starting hormones, medications, recreational drugs, illness. Often hair loss can be the first sign of a medical condition such as thyroid disorder or diabetes.

What is the treatment for telogen effluvium?

Identifying and eliminating the cause. Hair re-growth will then take a minimum of four months.

Celebrity client Anthea Turner, had a classic example of telogen effluvium combined with another condition, which in her case this was 'cosmetic trauma'. Anthea has always been known for her beautiful full hair, but she endured tremendous stress with the public breakdown of her marriage and moving house etc., which it all took its toll on her hair and image. "I have always been blessed with a full head of thick hair but due to the trials of life recently I started to notice my hair was breaking and becoming thinner. Following a consultation with Trichologist Sara Allison I started taking Hair Today More Tomorrow Multi & Omegas. My hair has now been restored to its former glory. It has definitely made a difference to my hair and skin and I feel more confident!"

COSMETIC TRAUMA

What is this?

Women do not like to admit to cosmetic abuse of their hair, but this is from over processing your hair i.e. practicing haircare at home or in the salon either incorrectly or too frequently, which results in hair loss or breakage. Mostly this cosmetic damage causes hair loss from breakage along the hair shaft rather than from the scalp and follicles, although this is certainly not always the case and can happen at the follicle too causing hair loss from its root.

What causes it?

- Chemical treatment of hair with dyes, bleaches, tinting, perms, relaxers or straighteners, which cause a breakdown in the protein structure of your hair.

- Over use of heat in styling practices, e.g, straightening irons, curling tongs, heated rollers, high heat setting on hair dryer and applying heat too close to your hair. The hair then becomes weaker, making them more susceptible to breakage which can then occur. Then even normal combing can lead to the sudden loss of hair.

- Brushing too vigorously with incorrect combs or brushes.

- Excessive touching of specific scalp area can cause 'massage alopecia'.

How does this happen?

1. Your hair shaft is 80-90% protein, the rest is moisture.

2. UV light, hair dye chemicals and heat, cause loss of this protein and moisture.

3. You get the protein loss a long time before you actually start to feel the cosmetic damage in your hair.

How should I brush or comb my hair?

There is the old wives' tale that says "brushing your hair 100 strokes before going to bed will keep it shiny!" This is false and brushing or combing should be kept to a minimum. Too much of it could cause damage and breakage to your hair.

However, because I am seeing ladies that are already experiencing hair loss, I find that some have actually stopped brushing their hair; therefore I do encourage them to at least brush daily to eliminate tangles. Be gentle and use either a wide toothed comb or a paddle brush.

Be very careful about the hairstyling practice of backcombing your hair and save it for special occasions only as if done frequently this can cause damage to your hair shafts and cause dull hair and spilt ends and breakage over time.

What should I do now?

The damage is being done even before you start to notice it, therefore I strongly encourage you to stop using heat on your hair NOW! Even before it becomes drier, brittle and breaks or before noticing hair loss. I appreciate how much women want to dye their hair and you won't want to stop until it's certain that this is what's causing you the problem, but please at least minimise the frequency, temperature and use the gentlest of products.

If I notice breakage, split ends dry or weak and damage hair what should I do?

- Stop the hair styling practices that you are doing and let it grow out for a while.
- See a good hairdresser for regular trims to remove any splits ends, as the longer you have them, the worse and higher up the hair shaft they get, then you won't be able to grow your hair with resulting breakage.
- Use a deep conditioning hair masque weekly.
- Minimise heat application.
- Minimise the frequency of hair dyes, e.g. bleaching, highlights and tints.
- Weekly deep conditioning with Hair Today More Tomorrow's Masque.

Alopecia Areata

Alopecia areata is one type of hair loss that typically causes patches of baldness. In some cases total baldness develops. In many cases the hair re- grows, typically after several months. In some cases, the hair loss is permanent. Treatments to promote hair re-growth work in many cases.

What is alopecia areata and who is affected?

Alopecia means loss of hair or baldness. The exact number of people affected by alopecia areata is not known but estimates are that 1% and 2% of people might be affected at some point in their life. It can occur at any age but most cases first develop in teenagers and children. In 60% of cases the first patch of hair loss develops before the age of 20 years and 66% of cases of alopecia areata are under 30. Males and females are equally affected.

What causes alopecia areata?

Alopecia areata is an auto-immune disease. The immune system makes white blood cells (lymphocytes) and antibodies to attack bacteria, viruses, and other 'germs'. If you have an auto- immune disease, your immune system 'mistakes' part or parts of your body as foreign. In people with alopecia areata, many white blood cells gather around the affected hair roots (hair follicles) which are mistaken as 'foreign'. This causes some mild inflammation which leads in some way to hairs becoming 'weak' falling out, which subsequently cause the bald patches.

It is not known why alopecia areata or other auto-immune diseases occur, but it is thought that something triggers the immune system to react against the body's own tissues. Possible triggers include: stress, nutritional deficiencies, viruses, infection, medicines, sunlight, or other environmental factors. There is also an inherited factor which makes some people more prone to auto-immune diseases. About one in five people with alopecia areata have a close relative who is also affected.

It is not known why it is common for only certain areas of the scalp to be affected, but these affected hair follicles are not permanently destroyed, they are capable of making normal hair again if the immune reaction goes and the situation returns to normal.

If you have alopecia areata you also have a slightly higher than average chance of developing other auto-immune diseases such as thyroid disorders, diabetes, or psoriasis. However, it is important to stress that most people do not develop any of these other conditions.

What are the symptoms of alopecia areata?

The typical pattern is for one or more bald patches to appear on the scalp. These tend to be round in shape, and about the size of a large coin and they develop quite quickly. A relative, friend, or hairdresser may be the first person to notice the bald patch or patches. Apart from the bald patch or patches, the scalp looks otherwise healthy. There is no redness, scaling, or scarring. Some people get a mild burning or itchy feeling on the bald patches. If you examine closely you may be able to see yellow dots, (empty follicles filled with sebum) or 'exclamation mark' hairs where the hair is narrower at the scalp, coiled hairs and black dots. The more of these signs seen the more active the phase is.

When a bald patch first develops, it is impossible to predict how it will progress. The following are the main ways it may progress.

- Quite often the bald patch or patches re-grow hair within a few months. If hair grows back it may not have its usual colour at first and looks grey or white for a while. The usual colour eventually returns after several months.

- Sometimes one or more bald patches develop a few weeks after the first one. The first bald patch can re-grow hair whilst a new bald patch is developing. It can then appear as if small bald patches rotate around different areas of the scalp over time.

- Sometimes several small bald patches develop and merge into a larger bald area.

- Patches of body hair, beard, eyebrows, or eyelashes may be affected in some cases.

- Large bald patches develop in some people. Some people lose all their scalp hair and this is called alopecia totalis.

- In a small number of cases, all scalp hair, body hair, beard, eyebrows, and eyelashes are lost and this is called alopecia universalis.

- The nails are affected in about one in five cases and become pitted or ridged. Unfortunately signs of nail pitting gives a less positive chance of recovery.

What is the general prognosis (outcome)?

- It is an unpredictable disease. Hair regrowth may be complete, partial, or non-existent.

- In many cases there are only one or two small bald patches which grow back within several months, and then there are no further recurrences.

- In some cases patchy baldness may come and go over many months or years. The size and duration of the bald patch or patches are quite variable. But if you have had previous episodes and hair has re-grown, then subsequent episodes are also more likely to result in re-growth.

- If less than half of your scalp is affected and you have no treatment, you have about a four in five chance of full hair re-growth within one year.

- With more extensive hair loss, there is less of a chance that hair will re-grow.

Unfortunately without treatment about one in five people who develop alopecia areata will progress to alopecia totalis (total scalp baldness) or alopecia universalis (loss of all scalp and body hair.) Progression to these more extensive types of hair loss is more common if:

- The onset occurs in childhood.
- The initial bout of hair loss affects more than half of your scalp.
- You have ophiasis (alopecia areata of the scalp margin).
- You have an atopic disease such as eczema.
- You have eyelash and/or eyebrow hair loss.
- You have a family history of alopecia areata.
- You have nail changes.
- You have Down's syndrome.
- You have another auto-immune disease.

Women often become extremely self-conscious, anxious or distressed by the appearance of this type of hair loss, however rest assured, that when I treat alopecia areata in my clients, it is very successful and complete re-growth usually occurs.

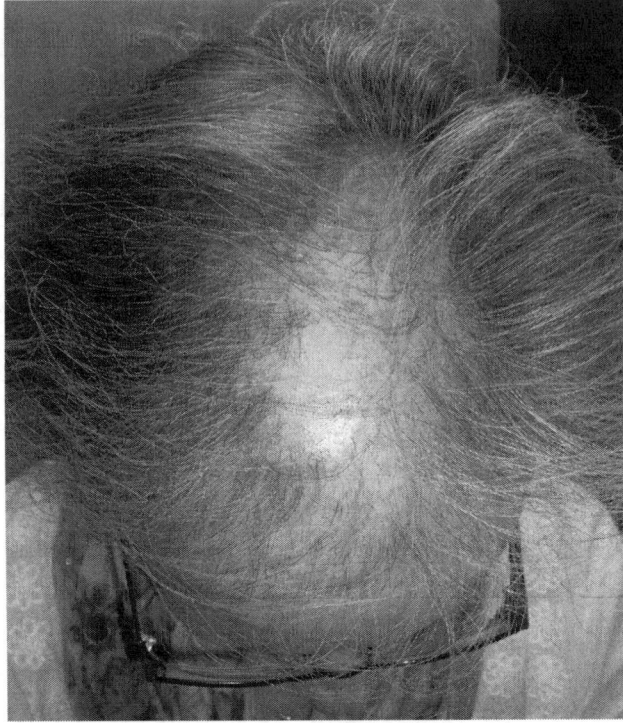

58 year old lady with decades of hair loss from extensive, prolonged alopecia areata.

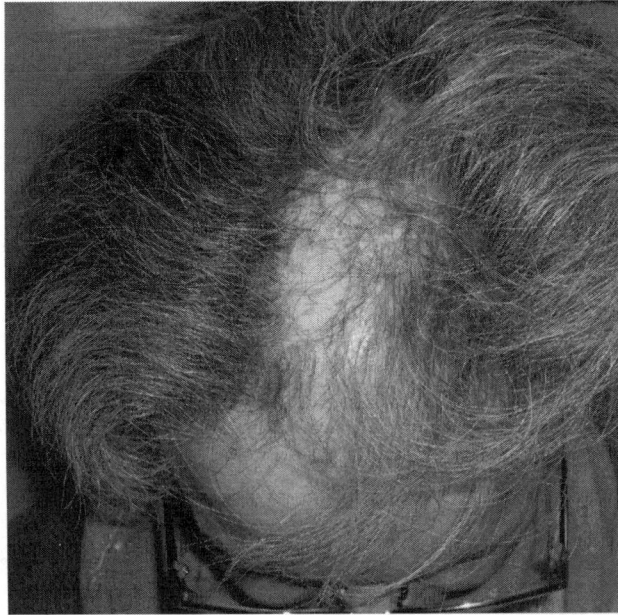

4 months post treatment, hair starting to thicken and fill up the gap,
note darker pigmentation too.

COMMON HAIR & SCALP CONDITIONS

Female Pattern Hair loss

Sometimes known as androgenic alopecia or AGA in women under 40 and senescent alopecia over 70. To promote a more positive outlook, I prefer to use refer to them all as female pattern hair loss and try not to use the word alopecia if possible as this is wrongly perceived to denote a permanent hair loss. However, this condition does not permanently damage the follicles, they are merely laying dormant.

Who gets female pattern hair loss?

It is likely to be first noticed at times of hormonal change e.g. starting or stopping of hormonal contraceptives like 'the pill', post natal or when approaching the menopause or early stages of starting the menopause when there are changes to the testosterone, progesterone and oestrogen ratio. This change can also cause increased facial hair and a loss of body hair.

- The American Academy of Dermatology research showed that 40% of women have visible signs of hair loss by the time they are forty.

- Ageing follicles contribute to the decline in quality, growth of hair and greying starts around the age of thirty five.

- By time a woman reaches her fifties as much as 50% of her hair has thinned.

- About 25% of women get advanced female pattern hair loss by age fifty.

- 13% of pre-menopausal women have female pattern hair loss.

- It is possible to see androgenic alopecia in children if they have abnormal androgen hormone levels.

Most women over fifty, who present with hair thinning, have female pattern hair loss, although not everyone has a predisposition towards this as you have to also inherit the genes too. Therefore someone else, somewhere in the family, either male or female should have also experienced this in the past. Female pattern hair loss is often made worse by telogen effluvium which is caused by other factors, such as low nutritional levels, stress or thyroid disorder.

What does the pattern look like?

Unlike men, women rarely go completely bald, they just get a diffuse thinning on the top and a recession at the temples but the fringe is often unaffected. Having fine hairs on 20% of your scalp is typical.

What causes female pattern hair loss?

Hair is made in hair follicles (the tiny pouches just under the skin surface). A hair normally grows from each follicle for about three years. They are then shed, and a new hair grows from the follicle. This cycle of hair growth, shedding, and new growth goes on throughout life. The following is thought to occur in women as they gradually lose hair.

- Affected hair follicles on the scalp gradually become smaller than normal. Sometimes this can happen rapidly not necessarily over many hair cycles. Oxidative stress can accelerate this condition.

- As the follicle shrinks, each new hair is thinner than the previous one. This is referred to as miniaturisation.

- Before falling out, each new hair grows for much less time than the normal three or so years.

- Eventually, all that remains is a much smaller hair follicle and a thin stump of hair that does not grow out to the skin surface, even though these follicles have retired, they can be returned to activity under the right stimulation!

Androgens are involved in causing these changes. It was traditionally thought to be caused by testosterone, but the real culprit being di-hydrotestosterone (DHT).

In the scalp at the hair follicle the testosterone is converted to DHT by an enzyme called alpha reductase. Only hair follicles that have receptors for DHT will be affected. These receptors are always found around the top of the head, not the sides or back (an important factor which enables effective hair transplants) Therefore it doesn't matter how much testosterone a woman has, she just needs to have some testosterone plus inherit the genetic component that makes her receptive to the conversion to DHT. However, genetic factors are uncertain and environmental factors predominate in late onset hair loss. The role of androgens, remains uncertain and deficiency rather than too much androgen may be a factor, especially in late onset hair loss.

Often the cause is 'multi factorial' i.e. a combination of many different elements.

What is the general prognosis?

Without treatment this condition is irreversible and hair loss is progressive. Therefore any treatment would be recommended long term for continuous effect. Treatment can usually prevent further hair loss, and often cause hair re-growth.

Female-pattern baldness is very similar to its male counterpart, although total baldness never occurs on the top like in men, women merely get a generalised thinning in this area and it can be extreme enough to expose the scalp quite plainly. Often the frontal hairline is maintained. As testosterone either low or high is a key element, women are generally of menopausal age when it is first noticed, however women with hormonal problems like polycystic ovaries can show signs of this from their late teens onwards.

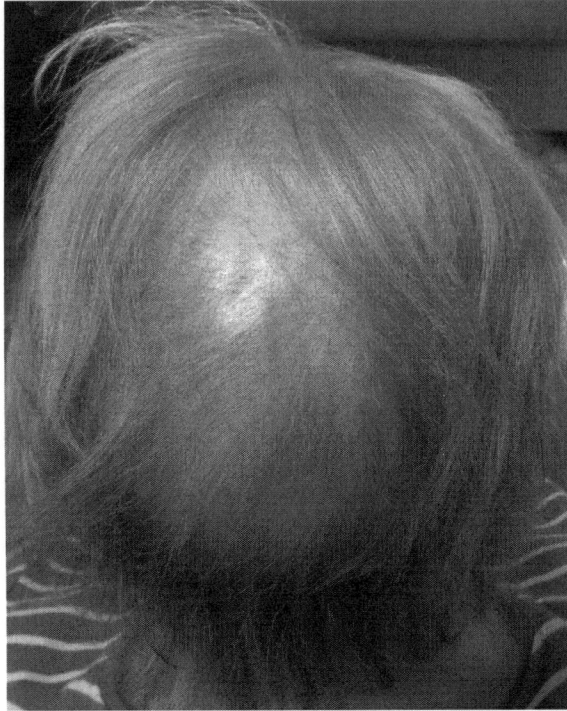

68 year old lady with female pattern hair loss for many years

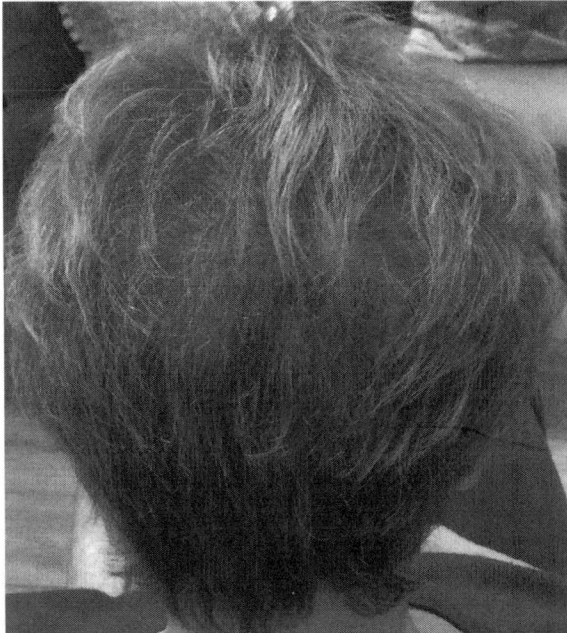

6 months after following her bespoke treatment plan

Frontal Fibrosing Alopecia

What is it?

It is an inflammatory condition that presents as a receding hairline in women, characterised by a band-like pattern of hair loss on the front and sides of the scalp. It's a progressive condition that appears as a receding hairline, similar in appearance to that in men, and can cause women to lose up to five inches of hair. The eyebrows are often thinned or may even be absent and there have been cases of associated eyelash and body hair loss, but these are rare. Unfortunately, frontal fibrosing alopecia is a form of scarring alopecia that means that the effected hair follicles are unlikely to recover. Average duration of progressive hair loss is just under three and a half years.

Who is affected?

Sometimes known as post-menopausal frontal fibrosing alopecia, it mostly affects post-menopausal women over the age of forty, although in some instances it has been known to occur before menopause and in men too, however these cases are rare. Cases tend to be in women from more affluent areas and in those who have other auto immune diseases.

What causes it?

The exact cause of frontal fibrosing alopecia is unknown. It is thought to be due to disturbed immune response (auto immunity) whereby the immune system attacks the hair follicles and where inflammation is a factor. This damages the stem cells within the follicle and if they are damaged, hair is unable to grow back. The skin in the affected area may look normal but is usually pale or mildly scarred. There may also be mild redness and inflammation around the hair follicles.

Frontal fibrosing alopecia may be a variant of lichen planopilaris, although this is disputed by some researchers. Lichen planopilaris results in bald patches on the scalp, and is associated with the more common skin condition lichen planus.

Frontal fibrosing alopecia first occurred in the 1980's, with more cases in the 1990's and in the past 10 years the incidence has grown very significantly! Indicating that environmental factors e.g heavy metals, pollutants/toxins are the cause rather than age, hormones or genetics. There have been some rare cases in men, but it is predominately females that are affected therefore theoretically it could be something in sun screen makeup or face creams e.g. SPF's. In a study 82.5% of cases used sun screen, but they didn't look at SPF's in foundations. I suspect it could be nanoparticles and aluminium contained in them, as only the organic products are without them. I therefore recommend trying Hair Today More Tomorrow, Rejuvenating Skin Cream, this special rose otto formula is blended with organic essential oils, which have natural perfumes, and a unique anti-ageing formula that will moisturise any complexion, including sensitive or problem skin.FREE FROM: artificial fragrances, SPF's, sulphates, parabens, SLS, animal cruelty.

In my experience with women presenting with frontal fibrosing alopecia Vitamin D deficiency does seem very common, but this could also be because of the use of sun screen blocking the UVB form producing vitamin D in the skin, therefore it may only consequential rather than the actual cause.

How is it diagnosed?

Diagnosis is usually verified by the presence of the typical whitish, scarred strip of hair loss at the hairline and possibly reddened, inflamed hair follicles. However, sometimes a scalp biopsy may be necessary.

What are the Symptoms?

FFA typically causes very little symptoms. In contrast to other forms of lichen planus, itch is frequently absent. Eyebrow hair loss occurs in 92% and can be one of the first symptoms and 25% experience this before any loss on head. The most common complaint is a receding hair line, frequently with inflammation around the hair line. Women can get 'orphaned' or lone hairs around the areas of baldness too. Loss of body hair can also occur. If you see red raised bumps around the follicles then this indicates that the condition is still active and progressive recession is usually about 1cm per month.

What is the general prognosis (outcome)?

Some people think there is little that can be done for FFA but this is not the case. While hair can never grow back from a follicle that's been scarred, the aim of any treatment is to prevent further hair loss and improve the rest of your hair. Treatment should be targeted for optimising nutrition, plus based around trying to control the inflammation which causes the damage to the hair follicle.

Oral steroids and anti-malarials have been used by dermatologist and it's possible these may temporarily slow the progression of hair loss, but they could have side effects such as depression, insomnia, abdominal pain, skin rashes and retina damage. And despite the assumed hormonal link, hormone replacement therapy and finasteride which is successful for male pattern hair loss has not been shown to be of any benefit. Therefore a hormonal link is doubtful.

Hair surgery is not a great option as you can lose the transplanted hairs, but is something you could discuss with a surgeon after 2 years of having a stabilised condition.

Traction Alopecia

What is Traction alopecia?

Sometimes also referred to as 'cosmetic traumatic alopecia' as this occurs when the hair has been held under prolonged tension by cosmetic practices like braiding, ponytails or if the individual has slept in rollers.

Traction causes hair to loosen from its follicular roots; however, hair loss also occurs as a result of inflammation of the follicles and their subsequent decline. If tension continues to be applied to the hair roots and the hair is constantly being pulled too tight in the same direction this can cause baldness to these specific, localised roots. Onset is gradual and often takes two to three years to become apparent and it often occurs symmetrically around the hairline in the front and temples. The back of the scalp is less likely to be involved. Vellus hairs which look like the small, short, fine hairs are usually spared in the affected area, so you may see these on the edges of the affected area.

If prolonged tension continues the hair follicle can become permanently scarred and destroyed, therefore they can get to the stage where they will not regrow under any circumstances hence chronic traction alopecia occurs which can then be described as a 'scarring cicatricial alopecia'. This results in permanent localised hair loss to those specific follicles under tension. Therefore it is important to recognise this condition while it is still reversible!

What is the mechanism behind it?

Three basic processes of traction alopecia have been proposed: trichotillomania, telogen conversion, and over processing. In all cases, immediately stopping whatever you're doing to cause it, can reverse the alopecia.

- Usually, the hair follicle can sustain trauma and still remain in the anagen growth phase.
- Excessive traction for prolonged periods, from tight braiding, wearing of ponytails etc; leads to conversion of the anagen/growing phase to the telogen/shedding phase, called telogen conversion.
- 'Hair casts' may surround many hairs just above the scalp surface.
- Typically, traction alopecia in the early stages involves affected hair follicles being pushed into the telogen/sheddding state, along with localised trauma to the hair follicles,
- Due to the hair shafts being forcibly pulled in the telogen phase, the hair follicle ceases to grow and localised alopecia results.

How common is Traction Alopecia?

The exact frequency of traction alopecia has yet to be documented, however it has been seen worldwide for hundreds of years as cultural, religious, fashion, customs and occupations have imposed an immense variety of physical stresses on human hair. The use of hair extensions, hair pieces and weave is extremely popular nowadays therefore traction alopecia is a common problem. Ironically women using these products do so to achieve the illusion of more hair and sometimes to camouflage baldness!

Which hair styling practices do I need to minimise/stop?

- Hair extensions.
- Styling your hair in a high tight ponytail.
- Hair pieces.
- Weaves.
- Scraping your hair back into a very tight bun.
- Extra weight from either long hair or wet hair, which can put even more strain on the hair when traction is applied, therefore can make alopecia even more likely.
- The use of rollers when applied too tight and repeatedly in the same areas.
- Wearing tight head scarves.
- Tight braiding of the hair into rows which may cause marginal alopecia and central alopecia with widening of the partings.

The resulting hair loss pattern entirely depends on your specific grooming practices.

Hairline

Otherwise known as marginal or alopecia linearis frontalis, this is a hair-loss pattern that usually results from the use of tight curlers, tight ponytails, braiding, weaves or straighteners. In this condition, the distribution of hair loss follows a characteristic pattern in the temples, starting around the ear area and extending forward in a triangular manner. For example, the constant contraction of the muscles used in facial expressions, in addition to the tension caused by braiding, may partially account for why this pattern is often seen at the temples. The involved area is approximately one to three cm in width in most cases.

Central

This can result from wearing your hair repeatedly in a bun. It is sometimes referred to as non marginal or chignon alopecia and is characterised by hair loss at the back of the scalp region where the bun rests. The typical client is a forty year old woman who initially complains of itching and dandruff localised to the back of her scalp. Similar to marginal alopecia, redness and hair casts can be seen on the scalp at the follicle. Sometimes, the front hairline may also be involved because the longest hair roots originate in this region, and these may be subjected to traction.

What are the signs and symptoms?

- Often asymptomatic.
- Hair loss usually in patchy areas.
- Scalp redness.
- Itching.
- Dandruff.
- Aching scalp.
- White hair casts/ scales can be seen sometimes on the scalp at the follicle.
- Pustules sometimes present.
- Broken hairs.
- Headache is possible if extensive pulling on the hair follicle is the cause.

How do you diagnose it?

It is possible to diagnose traction alopecia without laboratory testing. A qualified Trichologist can diagnose the condition by carrying out a physical examination and conducting a thorough consultation assessing repetitive use of hair styling techniques as outlined earlier and eliminating other types of alopecia.

What is the general prognosis (outcome)?

Traction alopecia may lead to permanent hair loss if it is undetected for a long time, however it is reversible in a few months if the hairstyling practice in question is discontinued.

TRICHOTILLOMANIA

What is it?

Trichotillomania causes traction alopecia specifically from the act of compulsive hair pulling, the urge to pull out one's own hair is irresistible and such an impulse can be overwhelming. It can be compared to other forms of self-harm.

It results in a patchy hair loss in the area of plucking. Once a hair root has been plucked several times it desensitises, just as when plucking eyebrows or leg and bikini-waxing. This explains why pulling sites get wider and wider as the feeling of relief is lost from the original area.

Hair pulling whilst it may appear a modern day problem with the young suffering the most, it has actually been around almost since the beginning of time as is even mentioned in the Bible, Old Testament (Job, Ezra 9, verse 3), and by Hippocrates circa four hundred years BC and in the ancient literature Homer in The Iliad. In religion, the Jain sects of India still require devotees to pull out every hair on their head to help them reach spiritual awareness via pain.

The term trichotillomania, was first used in 1889 by a French dermatologist Hallopeau, after encountering a young male patient who tore out every hair on his body in response to an intense itch.

Understanding the condition comes as a huge relief to the many people who suffer in secret, convinced they are alone and isolated.

Trichotillomania is a form of traction alopecia where hair loss is resulting from an individual repeatedly pulling out their own hair. People suffering from this, experience chronic urges to pull out the hair on their head, facial hair, eyebrows, eyelashes, pubic hair, nose hair and any other hair on their body. Bare patches where the hair was plucked will appear, and over time, permanent scarring and scalp damage may occur.

Who pulls their own hair?

It is a far more common condition than previously thought. Although statistics are scarce, it is believed to affect up to 2% of the population. Most sufferers are female, pulling is five to ten times more common in girls than boys and usually starts between the ages of nine and thirteen. However I have some elderly ladies that also have this condition, as it can go on throughout an entire lifetime or even start at an older age. By adulthood, approximately twelve females to every one male seek help for trichotillomania. In the United States the figures are similar, with one US study finding that as many as six out of every one thousand students developed trichotillomania. Fortunately many of them were able to stop again once exam stress was over. However, this condition belongs to a group of impulse control disorders; put simply "you don't want to pull but you can't help yourself".

Hair-pulling may provide a short-term distraction from immediate worries such as depression, anxiety, dependency or anger, but the pulling may then fuel a new cycle of all these feelings. It may create a vicious circle that is difficult to manage. Major life events such as an abusive home, bullying, divorce, chronic illness or death may trigger trichotillomania.

What is the cycle?

- An irresistible urge to pull hair.
- There is an increasing sense of tension immediately before pulling out the hair or when trying to resist an attack.
- There is pleasure, gratification or relief of tension when pulling.
- Pulling from more than one site on the body, can occur too.
- The length of an attack can vary greatly, with people pulling for anything from just a few minutes and a few hairs to severe episodes lasting hours or even the whole night stripping the scalp.
- Feeling of guilt afterwards.
- Recurrent pulling results in noticeable hair loss.
- Knowing that if stopped there would be a benefit, but they can't stop, so the cycle repeats itself.

What are the signs that someone has this?

Trichotillomania is often difficult to diagnose, due to the fact that some young adolescents are ashamed of their behaviour and try to hide it. And sometimes they just do it subconsciously, therefore are not aware of what they are doing. However there are visible signs that may indicate this problem. These include rituals like examining hair ends, twirling hair ends, eating hair, and running their hair along their lips.

What are the Triggers for hair pulling?

- Looking for hairs that feel different - thicker, coarser or wrong.
- Hair that is the "wrong colour".
- Ritualised pulling that continues until the "right" hair has been found or pulled.

What are the emotional consequences?

Many tend to hide their behaviour and suffer in isolation for years because of feelings of shame, hopelessness, embarrassment and depression.

The condition may affect a whole family, with the puller being the focus of much emotion and attention, much of it not entirely positive. Trichotillomania sufferers often report that their condition is not understood by either family members or the medical community.

What can you do about it?

Because it is an obsessive-compulsive behaviour, the best treatment is counselling to address the underlying psychological or emotional factors that are responsible for this form of self-harming. Therefore, cognitive behavioural therapy (CBT) or neuro-linguist programming (NLP) can be successful to treat the compulsion. Once the behaviour of pulling out one's hair is stopped, then provided that you can stop it in time, i.e. before permanent scarring of the follicles occur, then hair will regrow.

Scalp Seborrhoeic Dermatitis

Seborrheic dermatitis is like dandruff and sometimes you get a rash on other parts of the face and upper body too. It responds well to treatment; however the condition tends to recur, especially at times of stress.

What is seborrhoeic dermatitis and who gets it?

Seborrhoeic dermatitis is a type of skin inflammation, similar to eczema, but on the scalp. It mainly occurs in young adults and teenagers, but can happen at any age. It is slightly more common in men than women. Some babies have a similar condition that usually clears within a few months called cradle cap.

The exact cause is not known although a yeast germ, which is similar to a fungal germ, is involved. However, it is not just a simple skin infection and it is not contagious. This yeast germ lives in the oil of human skin (sebum), in most people it does no harm; but some seem to react to this germ and inflammation results. Therefore like eczema this reaction can be caused either by stress or by an allergic response to a product used, but most likely an intolerance to a food or drink that is consumed on a regular basis.

What are the symptoms of seborrhoeic dermatitis?

The areas of the body that tend to be affected are the ones with the most skin glands which make the sebum. Therefore the condition mainly affects the more greasy areas of the skin such as the scalp, the forehead, eyebrows, and the central parts of the face. Other areas which are sometimes affected are the front and back of the chest, the armpits, under breasts, and the groin.

- If the condition becomes worse a rash also develops. The rash looks like round or oval patches of red, scaly, greasy skin. Each patch is commonly a few centimetres across, but they vary in size. Yellow-brown crusts may form on the top of each patch. Several patches may develop which appear in a few areas of skin. The rash may be itchy and feel slightly raised as if it is on top of the skin. The scalp may become sore too. Some people also develop inflammation of the outer ear canal and/or of the eyelids.

- If it becomes severe then a red rash can affect much of the face, scalp, and neck. The condition usually persists long term and tends to flare up and down from time to time.

Why is this important to clear when I have hair loss?

The inflammation and flakiness on the scalp can cause blockage in the hair follicles and they need to be clear to be able to function efficiently and maintain a growth cycle for their optimum length of time. Often seborrhoeic dermatitis is a precursor to hair loss and excessive shedding can result, therefore it needs effective, early management.

What if it persists despite treatment?

The condition goes if the yeast germ is cleared from the skin. However, the sebum is a natural place for the yeast germ to live, so in many cases, the number of yeast germs gradually rises again after finishing a course of treatment and in many cases the condition tends to recur some weeks or months later. Each episode can be treated as it occurs, however, to prevent frequent episodes I would recommend using Hair Today More Tomorrow Sensitive Scalp Shampoo long term to prevent this condition from recurring.

Psoriasis

Scalp psoriasis can occur alone or in combination with psoriasis in other parts of the body. It looks like severe dandruff

What is psoriasis?

Psoriasis is a common, often heredity, skin condition. It is an auto immune condition which can be described as the immune system going into overdrive. The immune system makes white blood cells and antibodies to attack bacteria, viruses, and other 'germs'. If you have an auto-immune disease, your immune system 'mistakes' part or parts of your body as foreign.

It is not clear why this occurs, but people with psoriasis have a faster turnover of skin cells, i.e about every seven days instead of the usual twenty eight days. More skin cells are made which leads to a build-up of cells on the top layer. These form the 'flaky plaques' on the skin, or severe dandruff of the scalp.

There is also a slight change of the blood supply of the skin. This tends to cause some inflammation in the skin, which is why the skin underneath a patch of psoriasis is usually red.

What does it look like?

Areas of very red skin, covered by white scale. The look of psoriasis varies from one person to another; some have lots of scale and redness, whereas others have little of either.

Who gets psoriasis?

It has a tendency to run in families and affects around 2% of people at some stage in their life. It can first develop at any age, but it most commonly starts in your thirties.

What are the effects of having psoriasis?

The affected skin bleeds easily on scratching. Some people find psoriasis extremely itchy, while others have no discomfort. In some people it is mild with a few small patches being barely noticeable. In others there are patches of varying size all over the body. In many people it is somewhere between these two extremes. The severity varies greatly, with some days, weeks or months being worse than others.

Once you develop psoriasis it tends to 'come and go' throughout life and a 'flare-up' can occur at any time. The frequency of flare-ups varies and it is not uncommon to have long spells without the rash. However, in some cases the flare-ups occur often.

What is plaque psoriasis?

This is the most common form and is also the type that affects the scalp. Other common places are the front of the elbows and knees. The rash is made up of patches on the skin called plaques.

The extent of the rash varies between cases, and can vary from time to time in the same person. Many people have just a few small plaques when their psoriasis flares up. Others have a more widespread rash with large plaques. Sometimes, small plaques near each other merge to form large plaques.

Is there anything specific about scalp psoriasis?

Not really as although psoriasis can affect any part of the skin, the scalp is a common site. On the scalp, psoriasis usually stays within the hairline. Although, in severe cases there may be a solid cap extending beyond the hair margin. There may be patchy or diffuse scaling or alternatively thick asbestos scales. The crease of the ear is often affected and sometimes scaly areas can be seen in the ears.

What makes scalp psoriasis worse than having it on your face or body?

Because of the denser, thicker hair on your head, it makes it very difficult to apply lotions and creams and the build-up of scales can accumulate around the hair follicles. If left untreated scalp psoriasis can cause hair loss with increased shedding. If you treat it in time this can be reversed, but I have seen permanent scarring and hair loss occur in chronic cases.

What can induce a flare up?

There is no apparent reason why most flare-ups of psoriasis develop. However, psoriasis is more likely to flare up in certain situations, which include the following:

- Stress! It usually starts around the time of a stressful period, however once you have it, even though the stress may have gone, the psoriasis can be very persistent.

- Trauma to the skin.

- Many cases of psoriasis have been triggered by cosmetics, such as tints, perms or chemical straightening, therefore these should be avoided or at least avoid the more common aggravating ingredients, such as; PPD, ammonia, peroxide and resorcinol.

- Psoriasis may flare up if you have a feverish illness or infection.

- Medicines such as beta-blockers (propranolol, atenolol etc.), chloroquine, lithium, anti-inflammatory pain killers (ibuprofen, naproxen, diclofenac, etc.), sometimes trigger a flare-up of psoriasis. In some cases the psoriasis does not develop until the medication has been taken for weeks or months.

- Food intolerances can be a culprit, therefore experimenting with diet can be useful since a particular food might be stirring up the immune system. I would recommend IGG blood testing to identify any intolerance. However, gluten, casein in dairy, and alcohol are the most common causes of inflammation and intolerances for psoriasis.

- Vitamin D deficiency. Research has shown that lowered levels of vitamin D can be responsible for auto immune diseases, such as psoriasis.

What is the outcome?

There is no permanent cure for psoriasis. Treatments aim to control rather than cure and it tends to be more persistent than seborrhoeic dermatitis. As psoriasis tends to recur, you may need courses of treatment periodically throughout your life. Relapses are difficult to predict. I would recommend trying Hair Today More Tomorrow Extra Strength Scalp Shampoo which has exfoliating effects to clear the build up of scales, then applying our hair masque to your scalp and hair, because they will be very dry and will benefit from its moisturising effects.

Male Pattern Hair Loss

Also known as Androgenic Alopecia.

Yes this guide is for women, but not only can they sometimes have this condition, I have included it because my female clients often ask about their partners too, as after I have a consultation with a woman she then says "and is there anything that you can do to help my husband?". Their partners are sometimes there with them listening intently to see what they can pick up. I actually also see a lot of teenage boys and young men too, who even though they are grown up are often brought to me by their mums. Therefore I thought you'd like me to include this chapter too. Actually men can have several of the other conditions listed in this book too apart from female pattern hair loss and gynaecological issues of course.

What is male pattern hair loss?

Male pattern hair loss is the common type of hair loss that develops in most men at some stage. It usually takes fifteen to twenty years to go bald. However, some men go bald in less than five years. Typically, at first the hair begins to recede or thin at the front. At the same time, the hair usually becomes thin on the top of the head. A bald patch gradually develops in the middle of the scalp. The receding front and the bald patch on the top gradually enlarge and join together. A rim of hair is often left around the back and sides of the scalp. Rarely in some men, this rim of hair also thins and goes on to leave a completely bald scalp.

Who gets male pattern hair loss?

Nearly all men have some baldness by the time they are in their sixties. However, the age that hair loss starts is variable and about three in ten thirty year olds and half of fifty year olds are quite bald. You have to inherit the gene from some family member in order to be affected by this. Some women also develop a similar pattern of hair loss when they have large amounts of testosterone.

What causes male pattern hair loss?

Hair is made in hair follicles (the tiny pouches just under the skin surface). A hair normally grows from each follicle for about three years. They are then shed, and a new hair grows from the follicle. This cycle of hair growth, shedding, and new growth goes on throughout life. The following is thought to occur in men as they gradually go bald.

- Affected hair follicles on the scalp gradually become smaller than normal. Sometimes this can happen rapidly not necessarily over many hair cycles. Oxidative stress can accelerate this condition.

- As the follicle shrinks, each new hair is thinner than the previous one. This is referred to as miniaturisation.

- Before falling out, each new hair grows for much less time than the normal three years or so.

- Eventually, all that remains is a much smaller hair follicle and a thin stump of hair that does not grow out to the skin surface, even though these follicles have retired, they can be returned to activity under the right stimulation!

Male hormones are involved in causing these changes. It was traditionally thought to be caused by testosterone, but the real culprit is Di-hydrotestosterone often referred to as DHT.

In the scalp at the hair follicle the testosterone is converted to DHT by an enzyme called alpha reductase. Only hair follicles that have receptors for DHT will be affected. These receptors are always found around the top of the head, not the sides or back, which is an important factor that enables effective hair transplants. Therefore it doesn't matter how much testosterone a man has, he just needs to have some testosterone plus inherit the genetic component that that makes him receptive to the conversion to DHT.

Why can't men just accept hair loss?

Becoming gradually bald is a normal part of the ageing process for most men. No treatment is wanted or needed by many, however for some men, especially if they are younger or when it is occurring for the first time, they can find impending baldness extremely distressing and indeed even as much as for a woman! Men are typically more reserved when expressing their emotions, but I urge you not to trivialise the psychological effects of hair loss for a man when it is first occurring! Especially if the man in your life is your teenage son or a young man, give then lots of encouragement as treatment in these instances will be appropriate and when started in the early stages, i.e. when they still have a lot of hair, they can usually prevent further hair loss, and often get hair regrowth.

I would still advise a consultation for men, as similarly with women, there could be other contributing factors, and not necessarily simply male pattern hair loss.

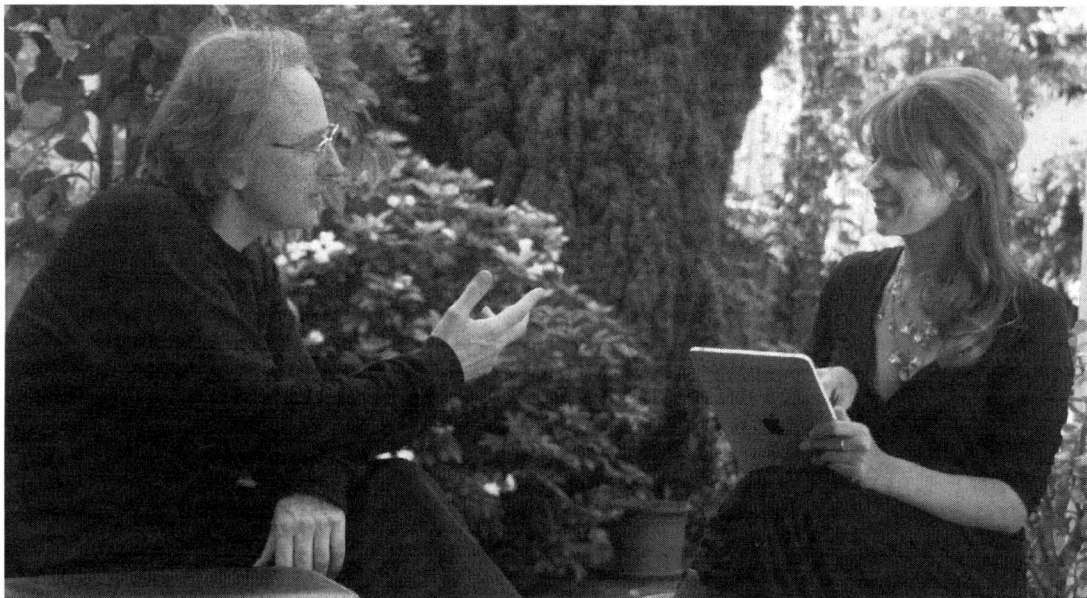

Sara consulting with a male client in her country practice.

CANCER, CHEMO AND HAIR

Quite often women will find the thought of hair loss whilst having treatment for cancer, the absolute worst thing about having the cancer! Fortunately this hair loss is only a temporary problem and this is just to guide you or your loved one through that difficult period.

Will treatment for cancer always cause hair loss?

There are many different types of chemotherapy treatments, which are usually prescribed according to the type of cancer and some of these chemotherapies impact hair more than others, some have no effect on hair at all. Doses can differ too and can therefore have varying affects anything from a little thinning to total baldness.

Why do some chemo treatments cause hair loss?

Chemo affects hair because essentially the therapy works by killing the cancer cells which are fast growing cells, unfortunately it can't differentiate between other fast growing cells such as hair follicles, gastro intestinal cells, blood cells, sperm production etc. The effect of the chemo causes a condition called anagen effluvium, i.e. it affects the hairs in the active growth phase of their cycle.

How long after treatment does the hair regrow?

The good news is that this is a completely reversible condition. Therefore, after your chemotherapy has finished, your hair will start re-growing, although it is likely to take four to six months.

Is hair the same when it grows back?

When hair regrows it can often be a different colour or texture or change from curly or straight. This is because of the changes that occur in the hair follicles as the chemotherapy alters the shape and size of the follicles and therefore the hair shafts that grow from the follicles come through differently; also the melanin production is altered and this will affecting the hair colour. However, this often all reverts back to your usual hair in time.

Should those who keep their hair avoid colouring their hair?

As you may be more sensitive at this time, then to be on the safe side I would advise against colouring hair, or at least use more natural or semi-permanent hair dyes.

How long after treatment can you wait before colouring hair again?

You can start colouring your hair again when it has at least a few centimetres growth, this is to be sure of the quality of your hair and then if it appears strong enough, it should be fine to proceed; however sometimes people can get excessive shedding after dyeing their hair and after chemotherapy you are likely to be more sensitive. Therefore, bear this in mind and avoid dyes containing ammonia, peroxide and PPD as they are most likely to cause reactions.

Do you recommend a particular type of hair dye?

The more natural the hair dye the less likely you would be to suffer a reaction and associated breakage or shedding, this will mean using a semi-permanent or temporary dye and making sure your hairdresser does a strand test as dye may take differently on your new hair. After about six months, your hair and scalp may be resilient enough to revert back to permanent dyes.

Can you take nutritional supplements when having chemo?

Yes, but many oncologists, unfortunately are not happy about their patients taking multi vitamins whilst having their cancer treatment, therefore you would need to check with your doctor first. There is a lot of research on vitamin D and cancer therefore if they don't allow a multi vitamin, ask your doctor at least about prescribing vitamin D if necessary. Even if you supplement or not I would still advise you follow my nutrition guidance, as it is vital to eat correctly at this time, especially when your appetite is likely to be very poor and you will require a more nutritionally dense diet.

ANTI-AGEING REVERSING GREY HAIR

Grey hair is a major source of anxiety for women at any age and one of the key reasons why you dye your hair is to disguise the grey roots. Often this can result in dry hair and breakage from over processing your hair.

Please note that age is no barrier to having great hair, I often hear women say "well it's my age, there's nothing you can do about it!" But this is simply not true, actually I have a strong focus on helping my clients regain their hair, by addressing anti-ageing, hence my signature product Hair Today More Tomorrow Multi & Omegas is formulated with very high levels of anti-oxidants which are important in fighting the ageing effects of free radicals. More about that later though…

Does grey hair really exist?

There is actually no such thing as grey hair, it is just a combination of normally pigmented hair mixed with white hairs. Hair turns white when the pigment cells at the base of the follicle response for colour cease to form. The pigmented cells are formed at the base of the follicle.

Dark haired people are thought to turn grey earlier but this is only because it is more obvious in brunettes than blondes.

Can you go grey overnight?

Scientifically it's impossible to turn grey overnight. Maybe rapid shedding of pigmented hair can occur, but even in the most extreme of cases it would take at least a few days. In alopecia areata (a condition that causes round patches of hair loss, but can lead to total hair loss). The grey hairs seem to be more resistant to shedding, therefore hair can look white and when it regrows often regrows completely white at the start.

When does it happen?

By the age of thirty most people have a few grey hairs and by the age of fifty at least half your hair will have turned grey. Premature greying is classified as occurring before the age of twenty. The temples usually grey first, then the crown and lastly the back.

What causes it?

Genetics, stress, nutritional and hormonal factors can influence hair pigmentation. Also some medical conditions will cause premature greying such as diabetes, thyroid problems and anaemia.

What is the oxidative stress effect?

Research shows that hair follicles are subject to oxidative stress which damages DNA and accelerates the ageing process. Oxidative stress can be caused by pollution, smoking, alcohol, vitamin deficiency and stress. Anti-oxidants can reverse this!

Why does your skin not lose its pigmentation then?

Research shows there is an enzyme present in skin and not in hair that may be responsible for skin not losing its pigment as you age.

Can nutrition reverse grey hair?

We know that stress (a cause of ageing) uses up vitamin B and some studies have shown that taking large doses of certain B vitamins, such as B6, B12 and folic acid have begun to reverse the process of greying in three months. However, the hairs revert to white when the vitamins are stopped. The hair follicle has a vitamin D follicle therefore it could reverse grey hair. Antioxidants are also vital and I regularly see my clients returning with significantly deeper and more vibrant colour to their hair, following taking Hair Today More Tomorrow Multi & Omegas which contains all these nutrient listed including a very high intake of anti-oxidants important for anti-ageing.

So what can you do to minimise ageing & grey hair.

- De-Stress as much as possible, with relaxation and regular exercise.
- Follow my separate advice on nutrition to eat healthily.
- Don't smoke, or take recreational drugs as these increase inflammation in your body, speeding up an earlier menopause and the ageing process.

- Minimise alcohol.

- Optimise your nutritional intake, by taking Hair Today More Tomorrow Multi & Omegas food supplement.

- Sleep well, try to get seven to eight hours per night, which is necessary for your body to regenerate.

- Don't pluck the grey hairs out! The old wives tale that you pull one grey hair out and two grow in its place is not true! But I still don't recommend plucking them as this can become addictive and compulsive and turn into the condition, trichotillomania.

Are there any other ageing effects on your hair?

As your follicles age they also produce less sebum, so your hair becomes drier and courser and your follicles can miniaturise so hair can become finer too.

Thinning hair can be seen in all ages, but as a woman matures it can become more prevalent not just because of her age but for these other factors most of which can unfortunately also can go hand in hand with age, such as medications, illness and stress.

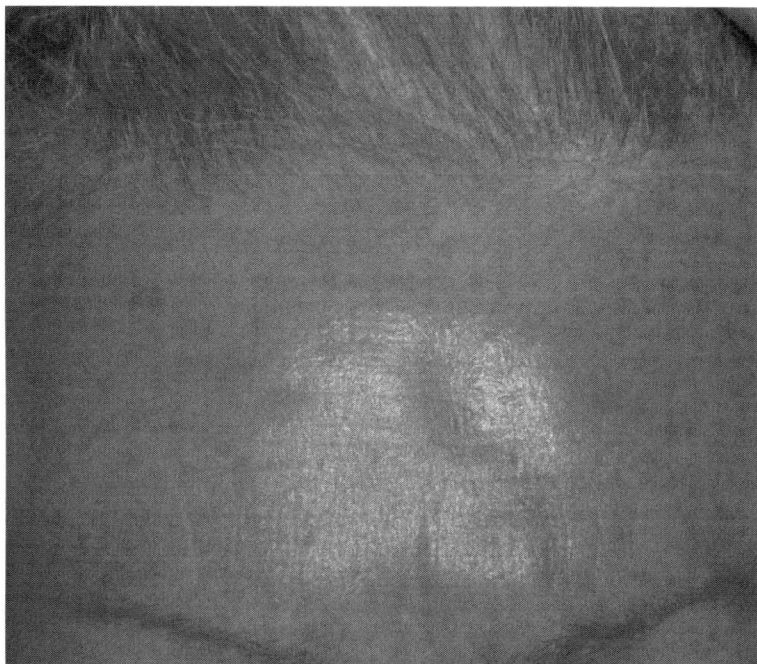

Before

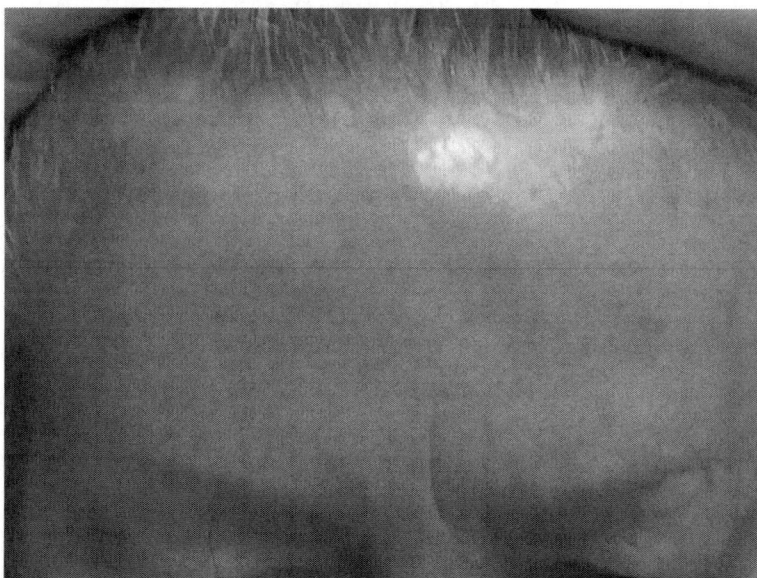

anti-ageing results for 69 year old lady after 6 months
on Hair Today More Tomorrow Multi & Omegas

HAIR NUTRITION ADVICE

Nutrition is something I feel very passionate about and the more I've studied it and seen its benefits on my clients, the more it has become a bigger part of my treatment for hair loss and indeed for anyone that just wants better hair. The advice here is applicable to benefit all the types of hair and scalp disorders mentioned in this guide. As a bonus whatever is good for your hair is also good for your skin and nails too.

Hair structure is 80-90% protein and this is dependent on proper nutrition to thrive.

Nutrients are carried in the blood vessels to feed your body and also to your hair follicles. These nutrients are essential for cell growth and protein structures that form your hair. If your diet is not rich enough in essential nutrients your body will use them up for your vital organs rather than for your hair which has the lowest priority in terms of function. Therefore, this can result in poorer quality and growth of hair and is an early indicator that there are issues in the body that need addressing. On the other side of the spectrum if you get optimum nutrition you can get such beneficial effects not only with your hair, but you can change your gene expression positively and can even reverse ageing and disease.

One of the biggest underlying causes of hair loss is from **inflammation** in the body and the hair follicles, therefore it is vital to reduce inflammation as much as possible. Two of the biggest dietary causes of inflammation are from gluten and casein, the latter being a protein found in 'A1' type **dairy products** (coming from cows), they have a common cross-reactant with each other, which means when you eat gluten and dairy together the combined inflammation effects are worse than if you were to eat them separately. Some people however don't seem to be affected; it's just worth reducing or eliminating them for a time to see if it makes a difference to you. Cow's milk is pro-inflammatory even without the gluten cross reaction, and many people are sensitive to this, so this is particularly important to avoid not only for hair loss, but also if you have any type of skin condition e.g. eczema, psoriasis or acne. Alternatively, you could try A2 type milk (goats or sheep) as these are anti-inflammatory and may give you less symptoms. You could also try other alternatives such as oat, rice, or almond milk. Dairy intolerant people can often eat yoghurt, butter and sometimes cheese, but sheep and goats version of these would be better tolerated even more. If you are drinking milk then ensure that it's the full fat kind!

Consider going **gluten free**. Many people are very sensitive even if not coeliac and it increases inflammation in your body. However, be mindful of processed gluten free products.

Don't smoke or take recreational drugs as these are anti-nutrients and increase inflammation in your body, speeding up an earlier menopause and the ageing process, including hair ageing, androgenic alopecia and grey hair. Research has shown this can be offset by anti-oxidants. Still best to quit smoking though!

Eat some **protein** at each meal. Have three meals a day. Vegans need to make sure they are food combining properly i.e. grains and pulses together to get the full quota of amino acids which are the building blocks of protein.

Half of what's on **your plate** should be non-root vegetables, one quarter protein and the other quarter starches carbs i.e. potatoes and other root veg, brown rice.

Quit refined **sugar** cane and artificial sweeteners as these cause oxidative stress, have inflammatory effects, can disrupt your hormones, are anti-nutrient and depleting particularly your valuable magnesium, which women tend to be deficient in anyway. They also have pro-ageing effects! Don't forget hidden sugars in processed food e.g. sauces, soups, cereals. Look for unsweetened alternatives or make your own. Xylitol or Stevia are good low GI alternative to sugar. Bear in mind, fat does not make you fat! Sugar does!

Regular and ideally daily, **bone broths** for its collagen promoting nutrients and if you suffer from IBS or gastro-oesophageal reflux, this is excellent for healing the gut lining With a healed gut lining, it's easier for your body to absorb nutrients.

Red meat two to three times weekly. Organic, grass fed and then cook at low temperatures to preserve the nutrients. The majority of menstruating women with hair loss have low iron levels and poor protein intake which are vital for hair growth, therefore this is a very important change I advise you to make to your diet. As long as you don't have any religious or moral objections, of course! I love and respect all animals and was previously a vegetarian/ Pescatarian for 20 years, so believe me, it's a hard one for me to admit, but eating organic red meat is more nutritious for your hair and your health.

Quit all **cola** drinks which contain so many negative ingredients, I could probably write a whole chapter on it, however fortunately it's not so commonly consumed by my clients. Still worth a mention for those of you that are still drinking it though, as it does contain, extremely toxic heavy metals e.g. cadmium. Cola is so acidic with the phosphoric acid that the body loses calcium, magnesium and zinc. This is particularly bad for bone mass in children and elderly.

Salt, excessive sodium chloride leads to increased inflammation. Switch to Himalayan salt as it contains many beneficial minerals.

Eat more **fibre**, e.g. vegetables, brown rice, flax seeds for bowel health and to encourage the absorption and elimination of toxins. You should be aiming to have your bowels opened, no less than once or more than three times daily.

Drink less **alcohol**. Alcohol creates hormonal imbalance and it's an 'anti-nutrient. In particular it depletes; B vitamins, vitamin A, zinc, magnesium, calcium and vitamin C, carotene. However, red wine contains beneficial antioxidants, it's just the alcohol that's a problem, therefore my recommendation is one small glass of red wine i.e.125 mls, with a meal no more than 5 times per week.

Eat more **Iron** rich foods, e.g beef, lamb, turkey, venison, sardines, seafood, eggs, bean & lentils, sesame seeds, pumpkin seeds, cherries, dark green leafy vegetables, prunes, dried apricots and beetroot. green vegetables, parsley, and thyme. Vitamin C foods taken at the same time will increase absorption of iron.

Reduce; spinach, rhubarb, tea, bran, fizzy drinks, antacids as these contain **oxalates and phytates** which block absorption of iron. Especially note spinach, as my clients often eat this daily, specifically to improve their iron intake and actually this can have the opposite effect, spinach in moderation though is fine just don't eat it for the iron.

Eat plenty of good fats as **essential fatty acids** are good for hair conditioning and hair growth. Include fish oils, flaxseeds, hemp seeds, olive oil, sunflower seeds, walnuts, pumpkin seeds, sesame seeds, borage seeds, grape seeds, avocados. Butter or coconut oil is best to cook with and olive oil is good only at lower temperatures.

Cut down on the 'bad fats' i.e. trans fats found in margarines, ready made meals, takeaways, crisps, chips, & other fried food.

Eat at least five to ten portions of fresh **fruit and vegetables** a day (one portion is roughly the size of a small apple). Eat fruit and vegetables in a rainbow of colours for their antioxidant pigments and carotenoids, e.g. green, purple, yellow, orange, white, red, and brown.

Snack on nuts and seeds, e.g. pumpkin, Brazil, almonds, cashew, macadamia, walnut, pecan, pine, pistachio.

Add two cups of **Epsom salts** to your bath before bed every night for three months or every other night for six months and lie in it for twenty minutes, this increases magnesium absorption. It is easier to absorb magnesium via the skin than orally. Magnesium is vital for relaxation of muscle tension, aids sleep, and relieves stress. It also aids with the balance of countless other minerals in your body. The sulphate which is the other component of Epsom salts is extremely helpful for detoxification, as it combines with toxic metals in particular and helps to eliminate them from your body.

Drink two to three litres of hydrating **fluids** e.g. spring, mineral or filtered water, herbal and green tea. Most of the clients I see with hair loss are dehydrated and not drinking enough fluids.

Reduce or better still eliminate **caffeine** found in; coffee, tea, cola and cocoa. Caffeine is 'anti-nutrient', it depletes your nutrients such as magnesium etc.

Reduce your intake of regular **tea and coffee** to one cup daily and not at the same time as a meal, as they contain tannins which deplete nutrients including iron, zinc, magnesium and copper. Coffee raises the ageing homocysteine levels. You should increase your water, herbal or green tea intake instead, as long as don't have more than three of the same type.

Dilute **fruit juices** 50:50 with water. It's ok to eat fruit, but don't juice it unless you dilute it, as it is too high in sugar and contains no fibre, therefore you could easily end up drinking too much fruit, vastly more than you would actually be able to eat. Blending is ok as you get the fibre too. But too much fibre can cause bowel problems.

Avoid artificial preservatives, colours, flavourings.

Eat **organic** fruit, vegetables, meat, poultry, diary and eggs where possible. This avoids the consumption of pesticides and is beneficial for animal welfare and greater nutritional value.

Avoid Junk food, as contains low nutritional value.

Incorporate my hair superfoods (next chapter) into your diet as much as possible!

HAIR SUPERFOODS

Superfoods are those that are very nutrient dense and I'm often asked by the media about which are good for your hair, therefore I just wanted to explain in fuller detail my two key hair superfoods…

Eggs

My number one food for hair! Eggs! Why? Well they have to be very nutritious as they are produced for the hen to feed it's chick for twenty one days, for it to develop from the size of a tiny embryo to hatching as a chick. Therefore this is the optimal time span for humans to eat unfertilised eggs before they start deteriorating. Egg yolks are full of nutrients that are beneficial for your hair including a great source of protein. However, an intolerance of egg whites is relatively common so don't eat these if you suspect you have a problem.

The egg is a rare food that has actually improved its nutritional composition over the past thirty years, rather than decreased. This is both due to the changes to hen feed and due to changes to ratio of egg yolk to egg white. Note there is a higher percentage of white to yellow in larger eggs. Therefore you may prefer to buy medium size. Eggs generally used to be smaller thirty years ago and the shells used to be thinner so these factors can also account for the change in nutritional values. The hens' diet changed from bone-meal and meat in 1980s to Soya and higher levels of vitamin supplementation in their feeds and additional enzymes that have been added have helped the hens have better digestion and absorb their nutrients.

Nutritional composition per medium sized egg:

Now 66 calories. Reduced by 15%

Fat reduced by 21%

Cholesterol reduced by 11%

No change in protein, but a value source and vital for hair growth and strength.

Contains omega 3 even if not an omega 3 specific egg.

Contains vitamin D up by 72%

Selenium up by 105 % to 12 ug per egg. A mineral important for hair growth and for thyroid hormone, plus a good antioxidant, both of which are of additional beneficial for hair.

Vitamin K.

Phosphorous.

Choline - as well as taking a role in hair growth it is also important in fat metabolism and has epigenetic effects.

Iron.

Vitamin A,

B Vitamins.

Calcium and long chain fatty acids.

B vitamins are important for energy release.

Therefore eggs are nutrient dense, so perfect for small appetites. Eggs for breakfast create satiety and decrease appetite for the following 24 hours, in particular for three hours afterwards. Therefore egg breakfasts enhance weight loss, but of course you can also have eggs at other meal times too. These studies were with three eggs per meal but it may be that two eggs have same satiety effect.

To maintain freshness and nutrient content keep your eggs in the fridge, but for best cooking results allow them to reach room temperature first, which usually takes thirty minutes.

Maybe you're still influenced by the bad press eggs had in the 1980's with the then UK health minster Edwina Curry scandal, in addition for many years people been told to limit their egg intake for cholesterol reasons, however since then there have been vast improvements to nutrition in eggs, which is mainly due to changes in hen feed and production. I strongly encourage you to buy organic eggs, for animal welfare reasons and for maximum nutrition.

Edwina Curry highlighted the issue about salmonella in eggs and now British lion eggs come from hens vaccinated against salmonella. Only 1-3% of eggs come from eggs that have salmonella known infected hens. All eggs in UK major supermarkets are red lion safe eggs. Just be wary when buying from twenty four hour corner shops that probably import from other EU counties, as these may be infected. Also be careful when ordering egg fried rice at restaurants where they keep the eggs at warm temperatures for long periods and then don't cook high enough or long enough to destroy the salmonella. Stress in hens can induce salmonella in their eggs which is another reason to get eggs from chickens that have freedom to roam and are well looked after.

Department of Health now say there is no limit on how many eggs you eat and indeed Edwina Curry now promotes egg consumption.

QUINOA.

Great for promoting hair regrowth, my second favourite hair superfood is Quinoa, (pronounced 'keen waa') which is a gluten free 'grain' and called the 'mother grain' because of it's sustaining properties. However, although known as a grain, quinoa is technically a seed. Like other seeds, it is rich in, vitamins and minerals, providing almost four times as much calcium as wheat, plus extra iron, B vitamins and vitamin E. Quinoa is also low in fat: the majority of its oil is polyunsaturated, providing essential fatty acids. Quinoa is also one of the highest protein sources in the vegetable kingdom, supplying ALL the amino acids including lysine which is usually only found in red meat. (Lower dose than animal products though) sixteen per cent of its calories are protein (soya has the most, at thirty eight per cent protein, and some other beans are also higher). Quinoa is easily found nowadays in the supermarket or health food store and can be used as an alternative to rice or pasta. Quinoa 'grains' are similar in texture to couscous, but a better alternative as couscous is wheat and contains gluten. Quinoa has a lower GL than rice and the GL load comes down even more if you serve it with protein, such as meat or fish.

Quinoa also comes in flakes' which you can make into porridge with goats or non-dairy milk for a healthy breakfast.

Other Hair Superfoods.

Being superfoods, they each have numerous qualities; I've only mentioned briefly my key ones.

- **Wheat grass**, for detoxing & eliminating heavy metals and to build, repair & maintain healthy hair follicle cells. Take daily wheatgrass shot. I recommend vegusjuices.com. *10% discount code SA1234.*

- **Green tea**, high in anti-oxidants, enhances fat metabolism and helps controls blood sugar, which are beneficial for weight loss. Green tea can reverse epigenetic changes. Theanine is the component in green tea that stops the caffeine from making you wired, it helps you focus and have a calm mind. Counts towards your daily fluid intake. Just be mindful it contains caffeine, even though in much smaller quantities than regular tea.

- **Broccoli**, for eliminating excess oestrogen and creating a better oestrogen/ progesterone ratio.

- **Ginger**, anti-inflammatory, anti-bacterial, great to drink it seeped in hot water or very flavoursome for adding to your cooking.

- **Curcumin/Turmeric**, epigenetic & anti-inflammatory, add to cooking and is more beneficial if combined with good fats.

- **Celery**, anti-inflammatory and for mood calming effects, therefore good for relieving anger or anxiety.

- **Beetroot**, a good non animal, source of iron, maybe troublesome if you have SIBO or IBS though.

- **Almonds**, for protein snacks.

- **Dark Chocolate**, high in magnesium which women tend to be very deficient in and could account for cravings for chocolate around menstruation when your bodys' needs are greater, it is high in anti-oxidants and helps you feel happier by promoting serotonin therefore good for depression & stress as it contains phenethylamine/ PEA which also has a satiety effect, therefore good at the end of meal to stop you feeling like you need to eat a huge sugary pudding. It does contain caffeine though so just be mindful to only eat a little piece!

- **Maca** hot chocolate makes a healthy drink, great for balancing your hormones.

- **Avocado**, high in fibre, essential fats, contains all the amino acids to form a complete protein (low dose), folate, vitamin E, magnesium.

- **Asparagus** for folic acid.

SURGICAL HAIR LOSS TREATMENTS

Hair surgery has improved a lot over the years, and whilst it's true I have referred some of my female clients for successful surgery, this option is usually more suitable for men. Women tend to have slightly diffuse hair thinning loss rather than actual bald areas; and surgery is better for the more extensive baldness such as for recession and thinning crowns in men. Hair surgeons typically turn away hundreds of thousands of enquiries from women even without seeing them, therefore if you feel this is something you are interested in I would advise a consultation with me to see what's appropriate for you, however, for most women surgery is just not necessary and I can help you regrow your hair naturally.

If you are suitable then the strip method often referred to as FUT, would be best because you wouldn't need to shave your head to have it performed. This is a skilled operation, therefore you need to see a good surgeon for best results.

Surgery could be used for your eyebrows and eyelashes. It is also possible to have surgery on scarring alopecia conditions such as frontal fibrosing alopecia if the condition has been stable for two years, however there is a risk that the transplant may not 'take' and may fall out up to a year later.

Does surgery give instant results?

No. It is follicles that are transplanted rather than the complete hair shaft, new hair growth from these follicles will only break through skin at three to four months after the procedure. However, it will take at least six to eight months for the new hair to make any significant cosmetic difference to your appearance. Sometimes, a result may take longer to show when transplanted over with scars or filling in a previously transplanted area. Hair continues to mature for over 12 months after surgery.

Will I regain a full head of hair?

Not literally. The surgeons are only redistributing your existing permanent hair to your thin or bald areas. They are not creating new hair. Having said that, in expert hands the limited donor hair available can be used to create the illusion of a lot more hair in people with significant hair loss. In extensive baldness, the most important achievement will be to restore frontal scalp hair and the hairline to create a frame around the face. This will improve how you look to yourself and to others.

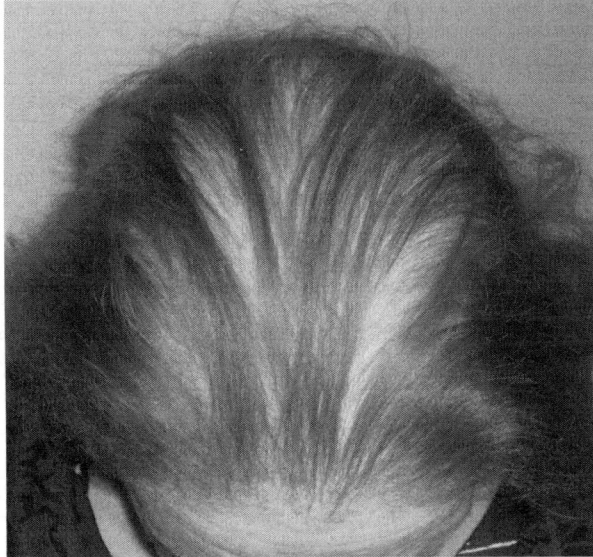

66 year old lady diffuse thinning for 3 years.

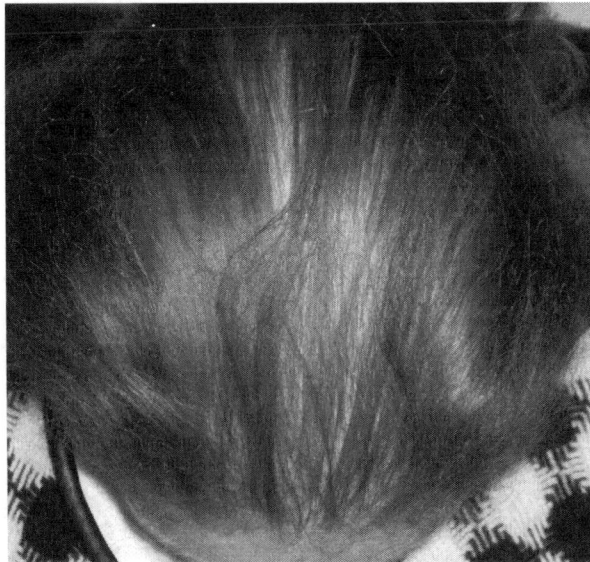

1 year post following her bespoke treatment plan.

HOW DO I FIX IT?

TOP 7 WAYS TO HELP STOP THINNING HAIR.

1. **Identify and treat any health issues**. Hair is a great marker for your overall health and well being, therefore if you are concerned that the condition or density of your hair has changed then you should see your doctor or qualified trichologist for appropriate blood tests and ensure you get any necessary treatment for underlying health or nutrition deficiencies that may be identified.

2. Be mindful of your **hair care/styling** routine and minimise damage by reducing the use of heat such as straighteners and blow drying on high heat, also be careful of over use of hair dyes and hair extensions and tight hair styles, as long term use could cause irreversible hair loss.

3. Nutrition is of paramount importance and in particular the hair shaft is approx 80-90 % **protein**, therefore to have good strong hair, always ensure you eat good quality protein at each meal time and eat 3 meals a day! Plus follow my other nutrition recommendations.

4. In addition to following my nutrition guide, I also recommend taking **Hair Today More Tomorrow Multi & Omegas**, then you can be sure that you are getting all of the important hair and anti-ageing nutrients in one single supplement. Not only will it help your hair, but you will also see vast anti-ageing improvements in your skin and stronger nails too.

5. **Increase your fluid intake** to assist with more hydrated and luxurious hair, aim for between two to three litres total fluid daily. Water should be a major component of your hair and most people just don't drink enough.

6. **Wash your hair daily** or at least alternate days. Many of my clients experiencing hair loss wash their hair less often this is the mistaken belief that just because they see more hair shedding when washing their hair, then that is the cause of the hair loss. However, it's actually more beneficial to wash your hair every day or at least every alternate day as this keeps your follicles and hair free from debris, bacteria and pollution. The only detrimental effects of washing more often is when you use excessive heat in styling your hair afterwards as this can be very damaging and cause

breakage. Just ensure you use good quality shampoos and conditioners, such as from the Hair Today More Tomorrow range.

7. **De-Stress as much as possible**. If you do have hair problems don't stress about it, just follow these simple steps;

- Exercise three to five times a week, i.e. at least thirty minutes and keep to it in moderation only as excessive exercise can be detrimental.
- Meditation, will lead to an emotional, physical and psychological balance.
- Balanced nutrition is another key to reducing stress levels. If your diet is rich in nutrients and vitamins, you will be less tired, more focused, and thus more capable of coping with stress.
- Regular massages.
- Stroking pets.
- Practising mindfulness.
- Physical intimacy.
- Spending time with 'quality' friends.
- Spend time in nature wherever possible.
- Relaxation technique.
- Seek help from a qualified professional if still stressed.

COMMON Q&A'S

How much hair loss is considered normal?

Hair shedding is a natural part of the normal hair growth cycle and it can be difficult for an individual to gauge what is excessive. But generally I would say if you notice an increase in your normal shedding pattern or if you see more of your scalp than previously you should seek advice. Quite often it's when you notice that your hair isn't keeping you as warm as it once was.

What are hair loss symptoms and signs

Tell tale signs to look out for would be seeing more hair shedding when washing your hair or when combing/brushing your hair, or seeing more lose hairs on your pillow or your pony tail getting thinner. Increased bad hair days, taking less time to dry your hair and loss of outer third or more of your eyebrows are all signs.

If you have lots of hair fall out after a shower, is this something to worry about? What could be causing it?

If you do notice an increase in the number of hair falling after a shower then this could mean you are having an abnormal loss. It's very easy to get very anxious when you see this, but it could just be a temporary situation. However, don't ignore it altogether as your hair is a great marker for your health and therefore you should seek professional guidance.

Is timing important – i.e will you see better results if you treat hair loss sooner rather than later?

Absolutely as it's easier and saves time, to hang onto hair that you have, rather than to regrow it after you've lost it!

Can your genes cause you to lose hair?

Yes, there is a strong genetic component to androgenic alopecia and alopecia aerata, both conditions can be caused by inheriting the gene from any male or female family members and can manifest in combination with hormonal changes. So if your parents, grandparents or siblings all have lovely thick hair, then it makes it less likely that you will have this genetic type of hair thinning. However, with good nutrition it is possible to 'switch off' this gene.

Do we get seasonal hair shedding?

Women often notice their own seasonal shedding that can occur at the same time every year, not necessarily just in Autumn. However, Swedish researchers found that women had the highest proportion of hairs resting in July and then 100 days later falling out from October onwards. Why this is I don't think anyone can categorically say for sure, but apparently some experts have said it could be an evolutionary thing where the body holds on to hair in the summer months to protect itself from sun damage to the skin.

How do environmental toxins affect the hair?

Environmental toxins such as pollution, heavy metals and chemicals etc., can cause oxidative stress and damage DNA which accelerates the ageing process and can potentially cause autoimmune hair loss conditions or other auto immune disorders such as hypothyroidism which can cause secondary hair loss.

What are the signs that your hair is in poor health?

Loss of lustre and lifeless, dryness, oiliness, less body and generalised hair thinning, but hair loss can also can show up more in certain weaker areas like the crown or front top, recession at the hair line or a wider parting.

Can our hair tell us if we've been eating the wrong things?

Nutrition is fundamental to hair health and gene expression. Therefore what we eat and what we don't eat can certainly show up in your hair appearance and display signs as mentioned above. Hair analysis can be performed at laboratories for all kinds of things including recreational drugs and heavy metals such as mercury.

Can lack of exercise or too much exercise have an impact on our hair?

Moderate exercise, such as; one hour three to five times weekly can be extremely beneficial for the elimination of the damaging stress hormone cortisol. Therefore if you are suffering from stress related hair loss this can relieve the symptoms. However, although most people don't do enough exercise, very occasionally some people do excessive, intensive exercising, such as; two hours a day or more and this can put the body under a lot of stress and actually create more demand for nutrient dense diet, especially more protein and if this isn't consumed it could cause hair loss as a result. When choosing an exercise to incorporate into your regime, ensure you choose a recreation that you enjoy or it will only add to your stress rather than relieving it.

Why is hair loss in women a growing problem?

Of course people are living longer and being more image conscious than before, therefore it is a bigger issue for those reasons, but also in modern society women lead more stressful lives. Plus in today's world we are more nutrition deficient than a hundred years ago. Even if women have perfect diets the way food is manufactured means there is less nutrition in the food. Due to being less physically active than our forebears women often go on crash diets to maintain their weight which can be detrimental. There is also the increased amount of environment toxins and of over processing, heat and dye, also traction alopecia with the popularity of hair extensions. A final reason is that women today have regular monthly menstruation instead of recurrent pregnancies and breast feeding throughout their reproductive lives which I believe can be a significant cause of low ferritin and related hair loss.

What age do women notice hair loss?

Thinning hair can be seen in all ages, but as a woman matures it can become more prevalent not just because of her age but for these other factors such as medications, illness and stress etc; most of which can unfortunately also can come hand in hand with getting older.

It's said that people can shed hair 100 days after a major shock. Is this true or a myth? Have you seen cases of women who have lost hair after trauma/stress/upheaval?

True! It can be normal to lose up to 100 hairs a day and when shocked or after trauma this can increase dramatically. There are primarily two conditions which are related to hair loss firstly alopecia areata which is often resulting from more extreme stress and can develop immediately, it is noticed in patches, but can develop to total hair loss. Secondly telogen effluvium which as a result of the change in the hair cycle is usually noticed around one hundred days after the event and manifests itself as generalised, diffuse excessive shedding.

Women often lose hair after childbirth. How can readers tell if this hair loss is 'normal' or needs treatment?

Hair loss after child birth should stop after around three to four months, if it continues then there may be other causes, that could have been brought on by childbirth like low ferritin levels from blood loss or pregnancy, induced hypothyroidism or maybe even stress from looking after a new born baby.

What effect can chemical hair dyes have on my scalp to cause hair loss?

If you have a scalp condition such as psoriasis or seborrhoeic dermatitis then this would cause your skins' naturally protective barrier to break down. This would make you very vulnerable to any products you might use, as they could then penetrate more easily through your skins' layers. Your scalp would therefore be more sensitive to chemical hair dyes which are quite potent and this could cause an allergic type reaction, such as burning sensation and swelling and hair loss! For anybody with a dry scalp condition my number one advice would be to wash your hair every day or alternate day, to help shed old skin cells; and ensure you apply conditioner or hair masque to your scalp, which will moisturise and aid restoration of your skins protective barrier.

So what effect can chemical hair dyes have directly on my hair?

Bleaching and dyeing can change hair structure, because the dyes and the bleaches used have to penetrate the cuticle (the outer layer of the hair) and get into the cortex (the inner body of the hair). Therefore repeated bleaching will significantly affect the hairs texture, it could leave permanently raised scales and upset the moisture content. It increases porosity of the hair and this makes further bleaching more difficult, as very porous hair bleaches badly, with uneven shading. Repeated bleaching leaves brittle hairs which have little shine or lustre and are vulnerable to damage, by weakening them, causing split ends and eventually hair breakage and loss.

Why does hair go green with chlorine after dyeing?

It is always associated with copper in some form and tends to affect repeatedly bleached hair. You will usually only notice this with blond hair as it wouldn't show up in brunettes or red heads so much. It may come from swimming pool water where chlorine or copper algaecides are used. Interestingly, it may also occur in the home if there are high levels of copper in the pipes. Green hair can even follow a long soak in a bath that has been cleaned with old bathroom cleaners containing high chloride levels; and very occasionally it is the result of using a bleach. Using a lemon juice or tomato ketchup rinse may improve the colour, but best to see an experienced hair colourist for advice and treatment. Don't worry it shouldn't cause hair loss.

Is it possible it's all in my mind and there is actually nothing wrong with my hair?

Absolutely! Some women are 'body dysmorphic' about their hair, i.e. they become excessively preoccupied by an imagined or 'minor' defect. This causes psychological distress, which can impair your work and social life, sometimes to the point of complete isolation. Therefore, my role can sometimes be simply just checking that everything is indeed all 'normal' and to give professional reassurance that you can trust!

YOUR NEXT STEPS

Will my hair grow back then?

As you have now read there are different conditions that may cause hair loss and some types are more reversible than others, but often with the correct diagnosis, identification and elimination of the cause and with appropriate hair loss treatment, your hair should regrow or at the least stabilise what you have and prevent further loss.

If someone sees a trichologist is it typically just one appointment required or a series of appointments?

Well this will differ according to the trichologist, unlike others Hair Today More Tomorrow take a lot of effort to prepare you with your tests in readiness for your first consultation, which not only provides accuracy of diagnosis and minimises your paid visits, but it also saves you valuable time and money. Because of the hair growth cycle it will usually take around four months to notice an improvement, therefore we usually only ask you to come for your first follow up after four to six months depending on the individual.

Is there a professional body for Trichologists?

The UK has the Institute of Trichologists, full members have the suffix MIT. There is also The World Trichology Society WTS and the European Hair Research Society EHRS, the latter of which consists of not only trichologists, but dermatologists, hair surgeons and hair research fellows. Sara G. Allison is a member of all three organisations.

What Products Can I Trust?

Hair Today More Tomorrow Multi & Omegas food supplement.

If you are unable to attend for consultation at Hair Today More Tomorrow then our Multi & Omegas are good first option and suitable for most women. These are vital even if you do follow my nutrition recommendations as it's so difficult to obtain what your body needs from the way food is produced in modern society. Bizarrely nutritionists say we are actually more nutritionally deficient than generations one hundred years ago.

It's important not to focus on just a few nutrients, but make sure you get a comprehensive range of them. You may be juggling multiple supplements or be confused about which ones are actually beneficial. Even with the best planning in the world, it would be very difficult to eat all of the nutrients necessary in a single day! That is where Hair Today More Tomorrow Multi & Omegas comes in, a complete product in one box! Developed by Sara G. Allison and scientists to specifically address the nutrition necessary to optimise your normal hair growth and with a strong focus on anti-ageing they contain all the valuable compounds that are contained within superfoods, including lutein, carotenoids, a full range of vitamins & minerals and more, also including; probiotics, Co-enzyme Q10, and extracts of Aronia berry and White tea – some of the most potent sources of antioxidants on the planet. It also contains a top quality linseed supplement to ensure you get your full complement of omega fatty acids. With Hair Today More Tomorrow Multi & Omegas, you can be sure that you are getting all of the important hair and anti-ageing nutrients in one single supplement. Not only will it help your hair, but you will also see vast anti-ageing improvements in your skin and stronger nails too.

The supplement works perfectly in combination with Hair Today More Tomorrow Rejuvenating Skin Cream which contains essential oils to help skin cell regeneration, the result is complete anti-ageing skin - inside and out.

Proven benefits from the nutrients contained in Hair Today More Tomorrow Multi & Omegas:

Maintenance of normal skin, hair, nails and bones, regulation of hormones, normal thyroid function, normal vision, iron metabolism, normal blood cell formulation, normal immune system function, normal mucous membranes. Contributes to normal skin and hair pigmentation, reduction in tiredness and fatigue, protection of DNA cells, proteins and lipids from oxidative damage. Contributes to normal carbohydrate metabolism, to normal fertility and reproduction, to normal cognitive function, to normal micronutrient metabolism, to normal fatty acid metabolism Contributes to normal protein and glycogen metabolism, normal amino acid synthesis and normal psychological function, normal formation of connective tissue. Contributes to normal testosterone and glucose levels in the blood.

Capsules or tablets?

Hair Today More Tomorrow Multi & Omegas capsules are a 'pure' supplement and unlike the vast majority of hair supplements they are free from unnecessary additives such as binders, fillers, colourings, excipients, disintegrates and diluents. You also need to avoid povidone (PVP) cellulose and modified starches. Sometimes all these detrimental additives can make up to 85% of the actual pill. Always choose capsules rather than tablets as the latter come in an impenetrable shell which is difficult to digest. The purer the ingredients the better your results!

Hair Today More Tomorrow, Extra Strength Scalp Shampoo

This has properties of anti-microbial, anti-inflammatory and anti-miotic (controls the over production of cells). This has a strong medicated perfume. The primary active ingredients are juniper tar, piroctone olamine.

Hair Today More Tomorrow, Sensitive Scalp Shampoo

Contains piroctone olamine and essential oils, It has a natural pleasant perfume and works as an antimicrobial.

Hair Today More Tomorrow Stimulating Shampoo

For those worried about hair loss, this contains menthol & peppermint essential oils which are known for their stimulating affect which can help lessen shedding. Really gentle on your hair; best used with our Stimulating Conditioner.

Hair Today More Tomorrow Stimulating Conditioner

Not only suitable if you are worried about hair loss and shedding, but also suitable if you have a sensitive scalp and fine hair too. Contains menthol & peppermint essential oils which are known for their stimulating affect which can help lessen shedding.

Hair Today More Tomorrow Intensive Conditioner.

If you have very dry, damaged and/or coloured hair then this is for you, it's a very rich conditioner containing olive oil and wheat amino proteins.

Hair Today More Tomorrow Masque.

Contains a blend of essential oils, this is a great treat for any hair and essential if you have dyed, processed, damaged or long hair as this will super condition it for you and it has a wonderful natural fragrance. Apply weekly to damp hair, leave for 1 hour then shampoo hair as usual.

Hair Today More Tomorrow, Rejuvenating Skin Cream.

With Rose Otto and Organic Essential Oils, for Sensitive and Problem Skin.

I helped thousands of women, with severe skin problems, feel beautiful and confident again by restoring their skin to its natural glow. My special rose otto formula is blended with organic essential oils, which have natural perfumes, and a unique anti-ageing formula that will moisturise any complexion, including sensitive or problem skin.

FREE FROM: artificial fragrances, sulphates, parabens, SLS, animal cruelty.

For best results use in conjunction with Hair Today More Tomorrow Multi & Omegas.

All Hair Today More Tomorrow products are made in Britain to highest quality control standards.

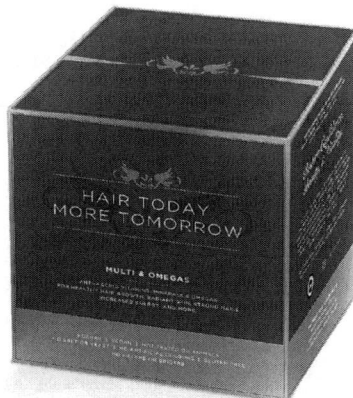

Hair Today More Tomorrow would love to further help you!

Please don't self-diagnose from this book, hair loss in women is a very complex issue with often multiple causes and I would urge you to seek professional advise.

Hair Today More Tomorrow is the first and only hair growth company with a unique **5-Step Hair Growth Support System™** that is shown to help thousands of women transform thinning hair into thick luscious locks.

Praised by Celebrities, Marie Claire, Prima, The Times, The Telegraph and more, all of our products and services have been carefully created by world-leading Harley Street Trichologist, Sara G. Allison, to reverse the effects of stress, poor nutrition, and ageing.

Unlike other methods, Hair Today, More Tomorrow products are easy to implement, painless to use, and made from the finest ingredients in the world.

Whether you struggle with thinning hair, hair loss, or just want to improve the quality of your hair, we can help.

To start restoring your hair AND your confidence today, call us now on **020 7299 0383.**

5-Step Hair Growth Support System™

Our process is simple:

1. **PREPARATION** Before coming to see us, we'll ask you to do a few small things, including going for a blood test so that we can fully understand what's going on inside your body as well as outside of it. We can write a letter for you to take to your doctor or you can use our affordable laboratory if you prefer.

2. **EXAMINATION** Performed during your 1.5 hour consultation with Sara G. Allison, she will analyse your blood results with her own unique professional interpretation. Plus under magnification examine your hair and scalp.

3. **CONSULTATION** During this consultation lasting up to 1.5 hours, Sara G Allison will take you through her extremely thorough and strategic history taking, which is a vital part of making your diagnosis and individual treatment. Counselling is given as necessary. After examination she will then make and explain your diagnosis, prognosis, treatment and answer your questions.

4. **IMPLEMENTATION** we will then provide you with your bespoke restoration plan that you can start immediately. This includes a customised Personal Treatment Plan and extra written information and advice to make your journey easy to understand. We'll support you as you implement our simple, painless, and discrete programme. It will be easy to work into your daily routine and you'll be able to start seeing results in yourself, your health and your hair.

5. **MEASUREMENT** We are so confident that our methods work, that we actually measure them. There are lots of ways to do this, but the most popular is taking before, during, and after photos that prove your progress.

PHILOSOPHY

We live by the following ethos to ensure that our services and products work:

1   SIMPLE TO IMPLEMENT – We know you don't have time to worry about hair loss, so we make things easy to add to your daily routine. You won't even need to think about it!

2   PAIN FREE – Who says, "no pain no gain"? Not only are our products and services pain free, but our products will actually help alleviate many of your symptoms.

3   DISCREET - We know hair loss can be embarrassing and stressful so all of our packaging is discreet. No one has to know but us.

4   RESTORE CONFIDENCE – We know your hair is linked to your femininity. We're positively opposed to scare tactics. We are here to get you results and make you feel healthy and increase your confidence!

5   COMPREHENSIVE – We don't believe in cutting corners. We do everything possible to ensure your success. You won't find a more complete and comprehensive programme anywhere in the world.

6   PROVEN – You are not alone. We have helped thousands of women, just like you, restore their hair and we look forward to helping you, too.

7   NATURAL – Our products are packed with the highest quality natural vitamins and minerals. If you're looking for the best, you've found it.

8   PERSONALISED – You're a person, not a number. We purposely have kept our consultancy small and create bespoke programmes so that we can meet your specific needs. Our only goal is helping you, not becoming a cold corporation.

9   SPEED – We are proud to say that our clients typically see dramatic improvements to hair growth and thickness in just weeks - 6 short months! So what are you waiting for? Get started today!

TESTIMONIALS:

"A great product" and one of the future beauty trends to look out for."
Times.

"It's all you need"
Telegraph

"Hair boosting nutritional supplements help with inside–out hair thickening. The latest testers report great results with Hair Today More Tomorrow"
Marie Claire

"When the balance of male / female hormones goes out of whack during menopause, a supplement might help regulate things. Try Hair Today More Tomorrow"
Prima

"I have always had a full head of thick hair, but due to the trials of life, I started to notice my hair was breaking and becoming thinner. I started taking Hair Today More Tomorrow. My hair has now been restored to its former glory. I feel more confident and I know the best is yet to come!'
Anthea Turner. Celebrity.

"I saw my hairdresser yesterday who said my hair has never been in better condition. Your product really works!
Sue Holderness - Celebrity

"Non-natural blondes know it's hard to achieve snap-resistant, lustrous locks post- bleach. So try Hair Today More Tomorrow".
YOU Magazine

Address: **10 Harley Street. London W1G 9PF. England.**
Telephone: **+44 20 7299 0383**
Email: **mail@hairlossconsultant.co.uk**

STATEMENT & DISCLAIMER:

This publication "How to keep your hair... a guide for women", contains information about hair loss and suggested restoration techniques. The information is not meant to constitute actual medical advice, and should not be treated as such.

You must not rely on the information in the book solely as an alternative to medical advice from an appropriately qualified professional. If you have any specific questions about any medical or specific dietary issues, you should consult an appropriately qualified medical professional or your own GP. If you have any concerns about your professional medical care or any medical condition, we advise you strongly to seek the further advice of your Doctor or GP. We do not accept any responsibility in relation to any self-diagnosis or self-medication or self-treatment using any of the information contained within this book, our website or our guides

If you think you may be suffering from any medical condition, you should seek immediate medical attention. You should never delay seeking medical advice, disregard any medical advice, or discontinue any medical treatment because of any information conveyed in this book, our website or guides.

To the maximum extent permitted by applicable law, we exclude all representations, warranties, undertakings and guarantees relating to the contents of this book. We do not represent, warrant, undertake or guarantee: that the information in the book is correct, accurate, complete or non-misleading; that the use of the guidance in the book will lead to any desired outcome or result; or in particular, that by using the guidance in the book you will definitely achieve hair growth or reversing or restorative effects. Your expectations should remain reasonable, as any and all results following our suggestions will depend entirely upon individual circumstances, age, health regimes, diet and physiology.

We will not be liable to you in respect of any special, indirect or consequential loss or damage whilst using any guidance or suggestions contained within this book, our website or guides. In this disclaimer, "we" "us" and "our" refer to Sara G Allison the author, on behalf of "Hair Today More Tomorrow Limited", a company registered in England and Wales under registration number 08198910, and which has its principal place of business at 10 Harley Street, London, W1G 9PF, United Kingdom.